Kirsten Hart's

BEAUTY

secrets

Dedication

This book is dedicated to every woman trying to look her best, and be the healthiest she can be. It starts when we're young and never ends. How we take care of our bodies determines how long we have to fulfill our purpose on this earth. Why not walk out our days in optimum health, while looking and feeling our best?

Enjoy the journey...

CONTENTS

THE CATFISH HOLE

A few months ago I was invited to be the guest speaker and soloist at a banquet. I have been asked to sing and share my story many times, but what made this time so memorable was that the banquet was being held at a restaurant called. The Catfish Hole. I was born in New York, and raised in New Jersey. Consequently, I can guarantee you: I had never stepped foot in a restaurant with the name .catfish. in it. Since moving to Northwest Arkansas, I have experienced many firsts, and going to The Catfish Hole was definitely one of them!

The Catfish Hole is located in Fayetteville, Arkansas, about an hour and a half drive from my home. It was a beautiful drive, and as I got closer to my destination, I chuckled thinking, "You know you've made it to the big time when you are appearing at The Catfish Hole. If my New Jersey friends could see me now....

When I arrived, I parked my car and went inside. The place was a dichotomy. There was a generous supply of overall-clad catfish lovers, as well as those attired in sparkly red to celebrate Valentine's Day, which was just around the corner.

I tried to follow my mother's rule for dressing for the occasion: always try to dress a notch above what you think your audience may be wearing. I was in a black pantsuit (my staple) with a hot pink sequin tank top under my jacket. Subtle black with a zing of fun. Not overly fancy, but definitely not overalls.

I found my assigned .speaker's seat,. and started sampling the homemade coleslaw and hush puppies that were dispersed on little white plates every two feet. (Gotta admit the hush puppies were really good.) Moments later my across-the-table-conversation-partner arrived. I introduced myself, and started the typical get-to-know-you questions: Have you lived here your whole life? Do you have any children? How old are they, etc.

When those same questions were directed toward me, I replied, "I have a son in college, and one that is a junior in high school." Before I could get another word out, my new acquaintance said, "You have a son in college? I can't believe it. You look so young! What is your secret?"

Well, I immediately knew I had just met my new best friend. Anyone that tells me I look young is automatically catapulted into the best friend club. It's not a hard club to get into; you just have to know the right passwords, and she nailed it. My new best friend's question caught me off guard. My secret? Did I have a secret? Before I knew it, these words came flowing out of my mouth. "Well, I'm happy."

There it was. Short and simple. Oh, I could have gone into so much more depth: skin care products I've used, exercise regimen, etc. But my main course of fried clams was being placed in front of me, and that was sufficient motivation to keep my answer brief. The meal before me prompted childhood memories of Howard Johnson's restaurants and the Clam Boat Sandwiches, minus the hot dog bun. I loved them. Brown clam strips, brown french fries, brown hush puppies, brown sweet tea, and greenish coleslaw. The dinner of champions.

The small talk continued, and I tried to include those catfish connoisseurs on the left and right also as we enjoyed the meal. They were sweet church folk. Some were also Razorback fans. The

Razorbacks were at the forefront of most of the conversations around the table. Following the meal I gathered my thoughts, spoke above the chatter of the other non-banquet diners in the restaurant, and shared my heart. After a forty-five minute presentation, the evening came to a close, and I started my winding mountain drive back home, which nearly lulled me to sleep.

A few days after The Catfish Hole experience, I happened onto a 14-day Bible study on my Bible app for my cell phone. There were various topical studies, but the one on wisdom caught my eye. Ever since my boys were babies, I always prayed for 'Godly parental wisdom'. Those exact words. My prayer was always for wisdom to raise my sons the way God wanted me to, with an extra dose of deep wisdom, please.

The study centered on Solomon's Proverbs. Whenever I think of Proverbs, the Proverbs 31 woman is the first thing that comes to mind —and not always in the most positive light. Don't get me wrong, the Proverbs 31 woman provides an example for every woman, but as a role model she's an awful lot to live up to. Seriously, who can compete with that woman?

Thus far I have never had the need nor the opportunity to collect wool and flax like the Proverbs 31 woman (although I've heard flax seed is wonderful for the digestive system—more on that later in the book). She brings her food from afar. I choose to bring my food from the nearest Super Walmart. She does not eat the bread of idleness. I am fairly addicted to bread. She also gets up while it is still night. I happen to believe it is unnatural to wake up before the sun, and preferably not before 8am.

See? I can't begin to fill her shoes. I don't know if I have the energy to be like her! None the less, I chose to read the Proverbs study. King Solomon. At least he wrote some pretty interesting verses in The Song of Solomon, which I remember giggling about when reading it in junior high.

The beginning of the study contained verses from I Kings chapter 3, where Solomon has a dream. He had just become King of Israel, and had offered 1,000 burnt offerings to God. God appeared to him in a dream, and told Solomon, *"Ask for whatever you want me to give you."*

Can I pause for a moment? Who, seriously, hasn't thought about what you would ask for if you could have anything you wanted? Wow. Imagine the possibilities!

Solomon, in his youthful wisdom, replied, *"You have shown great kindness to your servant, my father David, because he was faithful to you and righteous and upright in heart. You have continued this great kindness to him and have given him a son to sit on his throne this very day. Now, O Lord my God, you have made your servant king in place of my father David. But I am only a little child and do not know how to carry out my duties. Your servant is here among the people you have chosen, a great people, too numerous to count or number. So give your servant a discerning heart to govern your people and to distinguish between right and wrong. For who is able to govern this great people of yours?"*

I have to admit that my request would probably have been different than that of Solomon. Perhaps a Caribbean Island. Unlimited prosperity and health for my whole family would also have been at the top of the list. Solomon asked for wisdom. It's a good thing. He was wise even before God granted his wish.

"The Lord was pleased that Solomon had asked for this. So God said to him, "Since you have asked for this and not for long life or wealth for yourself, nor have asked for the death of your enemies but for discernment in administering justice, I will do what you have asked. I will give you a wise and discerning heart, so that there will never have been anyone like you, nor will there ever be. Moreover, I will give you what you have not asked for—both riches and honor — so that in your lifetime you

will have no equal among kings. And if you walk in my ways and obey my statutes and commands as David your father did, I will give you a long life.'"

I think we can all learn from that passage. If God ever appears to me in a dream, and tells me to ask for whatever I want, I need to ask for something pertaining to wisdom. It's unbelievable that God then tells Solomon that because he didn't ask for something selfish in nature, that He would be given riches and wisdom that no man before nor after would ever attain. Now that's a good dream. When Solomon woke up, it all came to pass.

The wisdom and wealth of Solomon has been recorded and recognized for centuries. No man has even come close. So since God was the One who gave Solomon his wisdom, we can trust that his words are true. Godly wisdom...God-given wisdom. Wise for me to follow because Solomon was the wisest of any man that has ever lived.

Even though the Bible study was a 14-day study, I read the first three days' worth of readings in my first sitting. I know; I should have paced myself. Some regard this as being an overachiever. However, each day's reading was only a few verses long. Three days' worth only took me about ten minutes.

With a good start on the Bible study it was time

to get some work done. I had started the project of repainting a room to become our new master bedroom. I am a tad ADD when it comes to projects around the house. A little here...a little there. Get laundry going. Paint a bit. Clean a toilet. Paint some more. Get dinner going. Paint. Eventually, everything gets done. It may take a little longer my way, but I have a system (most of the time).

I was rather proud of myself that I had finished three days' worth of the new devotional study. I was also fairly proud that I had finished painting the upper trim. Upper trim can be taxing on the arms. No breaks, and the arms can feel that pain for days. I had selected Ralph Lauren Soft Gold paint, which was starting to dry, and I was feeling a mini break approaching.

See. I am so not the Proverbs 31 woman. She would have stuck with the painting till it was complete. She also probably would have been wearing scarlet or purple linens instead of manly-looking sweats. There's so much to live up to when you compare yourself to the Proverbs 31 woman.

Feeling a sense of accomplishment, I took a break to read the next day's devotional. I sat on the painting drop cloth, and read day four. Day four had a great verse. Proverbs 3:21 (The Message version).

"Dear friend, guard Clear Thinking and Common Sense with your life; don't for a minute lose sight of them. They'll keep your soul alive and well, they'll keep you fit and attractive."

I re-read the verse. Fit and attractive? What? A promise that will make you attractive? How have I missed this verse my whole life? So if I seek after clear thinking and common sense, I can be in shape and look good? This was amazing.

I began to ponder what other hidden secrets Solomon had written about, and how I had not seen this before? I wondered about my comment at The Catfish House. My 'secret' to looking so young, "I'm happy." I wondered if that was a biblical truth. Could being happy actually make you look younger? Was there a hidden verse of wisdom to prove that thought truthful?

I decided that my painting was done for the afternoon. I had a new quest: I would finish the fourteen day study that afternoon. I was on a new found journey to search out what else the Bible could tell me about being fit and attractive. What woman doesn't want to look her best? The beauty industry is a multi-billion dollar industry. Have I been searching for the perfect wrinkle cream when all along the answers where right within my Bible?

My study that afternoon was the foundation for this book. I truly do believe that you won't need any more Beauty Secrets books. You'll be amazed at what God's word says about being healthy and staying young.

Perhaps you'll think of me when someone asks you, "What's your secret to looking so young?" And if we ever have the privilege of meeting in person, and you ask me that same question, you will automatically become my new best friend!

CREDENTIALS?

You may wonder, "What credentials does Kirsten have to write a book about beauty secrets?' That's a great question. I would probably ask the same thing. I'm not a supermodel, although I did attend the Barbizon School of Modeling in 1984. I can't believe my parents (thank you mom and dad) paid all that money so that I could learn to walk to the end of a runway, and pivot with both hands on my waist. I do get a few credential points for turning around and teaching at a Barbizon School of Modeling in 1989. Those poor girls (and few guys) that I taught. At least they learned how to properly apply blue eye shadow.

I am not a fitness guru, either. So much of physical beauty is rooted in our health, fitness, and the foods we eat. To be honest with you, there is at this present moment a chocolate-chip chocolate cake sitting on my kitchen counter that has been calling to me all morning. And I, with my acute hearing abilities, have been listening to it. That will cost me some extra minutes on the elliptical machine later this afternoon.

I will claim age as a credential. At the age of forty-eight, I finally feel as though I have lived enough years to know a few things about a lot of topics. I remember being a mother of two in my twenties (I had our first son at twenty six). Being in my twenties, whenever someone would ask me my age and I replied, I heard so many, "Oh, you're still such a baby" comments. Couldn't stand them. I was not a baby. I was a mother of two boys. Turning thirty was a glorious day. No longer did people refer to me as being so young. I had turned the corner into womanhood. Loved it. I love being forty-eight even more so. I am less than two years away from being half-way through my life. I fully intend to live to the age of 100, as long as my mind and bodily functions are intact and functioning.

I'm not sure if I can claim this as a credential or not, but when I substitute teach in high schools I have had hall monitor teachers say, "Hurry up to your class or you are going to be late!" Now, those may seem like simple words, but to a woman in her forties, you may as well have told me that I could eat unlimited calories without gaining a pound. Yes, it was that wonderful to hear. Keep yelling at me hall monitors...you are just making my day! To be mistaken for a high school student—yup, I believe that could be a Beauty Secrets author credential! I guess I should mention that some of those teachers may have been older than dirt and partially blind, but a compliment. is a compliment. I'll take 'em where I can get 'em.

I have read countless fashion magazine articles and books on beauty and health. I have watched afternoon talk shows chock full of tips and tricks to looking and feeling younger. I have worked as a fragrance model. Yes, the people that spray perfume into the air, and on you. (Not sure that last one counts as anything, but I sure got a lot of free cologne from those days.) I have sought after ways to preserve my skin and prevent future skin damage. I have tried every diet from the Cabbage Soup Diet to the (I almost died of lack of bread and just wanted a simple bowl of cereal) No Carbs Diet. I have finally come to a marvelous conclusion. Live life in moderation. Be wise about your choices, and live life to the fullest. Be joyful, smile, and appreciate every day you are given. Seek wisdom, and find answers.

It is interesting to see two schools of thought when it comes to beauty, for I believe there are two extremes. Some emphasize that true beauty is only on the inside. Do not be concerned with what is on the outside; just concentrate on your inner beauty. The opposite is the thought that we are what people see. People will judge us by our physical appearance, and that is of utmost importance. Face first: first impressions last. To be successful, you must look the part on the outside. I, personally, believe there are truths found with both viewpoints.

Audrey Hepburn, considered by many to be one of the most physically beautiful women in the twentieth century had such wise words about beauty.

"For Attractive lips, speak words of kindness. For lovely eyes, seek out the good in people. For a slim figure, share your food with the hungry. For beautiful hair, let a child run their fingers through it once a day. For poise, walk with the knowledge that you never walk alone. People, more than things, have to be restored, renewed, revived, reclaimed, and redeemed.

Remember, if you ever need a helping hand, you will find one at the end of each of your arms. As you grow older, you will discover that you have two hands, one for helping yourself and the other for helping others."

"I believe in pink. I believe that laughing is the best calorie burner. I believe in kissing, kissing a lot. I believe in being strong when everything seems to be going wrong. I believe that happy girls are the prettiest girls. I believe that tomorrow is another day and I believe in miracles."

Those are great words. Inner beauty reflecting to create outer beauty. That's wisdom. Audrey Hepburn took care of her skin, wore make-up and fashionable clothes, but her inner beauty is what radiated through her outer layer. When we women find the right balance of taking care of our soul and spirit, eating properly for optimum health, find the right balance of exercise, learn proven techniques for taking care of our skin, then we are living life at our fullest. Doesn't every woman want to be as beautiful as we can? I know I do. I want to look my best for my husband and my sons. I also want to love from such a deep place, that my inner beauty and love oozes out.

My beauty expert credentials may be sketchy, but like Solomon, I have yearned for wisdom. "*Ask and it will be given to you: seek and you will find: knock and the door will be opened to you.*" (Matthew 7:7) It is my desire that you live at 100% of your potential, and I have prayed for wisdom so I can share important keys with you to help you reach your full potential. I believe that includes walking in God's ways and living the life God has fashioned for you so that you can be the healthiest you possible.

If you are married, may your husband look at you with admiration for the beautiful woman God gave him. If you are a mother, may your children rise up and call you blessed. If you're not married yet, may the words and insight shared in this book help reveal the beautiful you within so that your future Prince Charming will be utterly smitten with your radiant beauty! To every reader: may you live each day full of joy, peace, and happiness.

SOLOMON'S BEAUTY TIPS

Are you ready to begin? Do you want some of these secrets? Here we go. I want to begin by looking at some verses in Proverbs. Again, the wisest man ever (God said so) wrote these words. These secret gems are chock full of priceless information. If applied, I believe they will change your life. I'm so excited to share these words with you!

"Dear friend, guard Clear Thinking and Common Sense with your life; don't for a minute lose sight of them. They'll keep your soul alive and well, they'll keep you fit and attractive." — Proverbs 3:21-22

I know I shared this portion of Proverbs 3 earlier. It's worth repeating. What an amazing promise! Proverbs' main character is Lady Wisdom.

Lady Wisdom was always kind of odd to me. Is she an actual person? After studying how scholars decipher Lady Wisdom, 'she' is a personification of wisdom; the wisdom of God, his ways, and laws. Wisdom is the foundation of all general revelation—what can be known about God and his law from observing the universe around us...a tad bit confusing, I know.

Clear Thinking and Common Sense are also personifications, but are exactly what their names signify: a little easier to understand. To guard clear thinking and common sense seem, well, common sense. Clear thinking: reasoning unclouded by biases, prejudices, hopes and fears, and uncritically accepted assumptions or facts. The official definition of common sense is: sound and prudent judgment based on a simple perception of the situation or facts. Fancy words,

I know. Basically, think clearly and do what you know is right. Proverbs 3:21-22 gives us the promise that if we guard common thinking and common sense, in correlation to God's laws and principles, that we are able to attain a soul that is alive and well, and we will be fit and attractive.

Some may debate that the word attractive here refers to inner beauty alone. The portion of scripture is taken from The Message version of the Bible. If you are a King James only version reader, that portion of scripture reads: *"My son, let not them depart from thine eyes: keep sound wisdom and discretion: So shall they be life unto thy soul, and grace to thy neck."* Granted, the words 'grace to thy neck.' and 'attractiveness' seem a bit different. I love The Message version. Since this book is about beauty, and not scriptural interpretation of different Bible versions, I have chosen to stick with the wisdom and research of the author of The Message version. Feel free to read the future passages referred to in this book in whatever Bible version you prefer. But, if you wouldn't mind, I will continue to quote from The Message. I happen to like the interpretation that mentions attractiveness.

Americans literally spend hundreds of BILLIONS of dollars a year on the quest for personal fitness. I have contributed to that amount. Perhaps not in the billions, personally, but definitely hundreds and hundreds of dollars. We have a family gym membership that is a little over $30 a month (which is actually extremely inexpensive compared to many athletic clubs and gyms). I spend cash on energy bars, weight loss pills, workout clothes, special foods and cereals that are advertised as low in caloric value. The goal of physical fitness is a determining factor in our everyday lives.

Proverbs 3:22 states that guarding Clear

Thinking and Common Sense will keep you physically fit. What a promise. What a possibility! Guarding has responsibility, though. Is it clear thinking to gorge yourself on fattening foods? No. Is it common sense to eat enormous amounts of food? No. That's where the word moderation comes into play. We will study more about food consumption wisdom later in the book. It's important. It's life changing.

Siren Magazine estimated that American women spend an average of $12,000 annually on beauty and grooming products. Unreal isn't it! That amount includes spa treatments, haircuts, cosmetics, hair products, perfumes, etc. The amount is staggering. Honestly, I'm so frugal that I don't think I come close to that amount. At least I hope I don't. I've never added up receipts from all of my purchases. Now I don't want to. I have a feeling it would make me sick to my stomach to see how much I spend on personal products. I'm not going to give up buying make-up and beauty products, but I want to incorporate as much clear thinking and common sense as I can. After all, King Solomon promises attractiveness. An impressive promise! "*You'll travel safely; you'll neither tire nor trip. You'll take afternoon naps without a worry; you'll enjoy a good night's sleep.*" Proverbs 3: 23-24. These two verses are right up my alley. I love to sleep. I'm not ashamed to admit it. I LOVE SLEEPING. There, I said it. According to statistics, about 40 million people in the United States suffer from chronic long-term sleep disorders each year and an additional 20 million people experience occasional sleep problems. These are staggering numbers.

My husband and I are blessed. And I don't take it lightly that we enjoy solid sleep without any disorders or having to take sleeping pills. Don't get me wrong: if you suffer from sleep disorders, I'm not saying you are not guarding Clear Thinking and Common Sense with your life.

There are actual chemical disorders that cause sleeplessness. I'm just quoting Proverbs 3:24. Who doesn't want to enjoy a good night's sleep'?

The Mayo Clinic recommends that adults should have between 7-10 hours of sleep a night. There are so many health and beauty benefits to a good night's sleep. More to come in later chapters! Beauty sleep isn't just a myth, it's a necessity. You'll be surprised how necessary it is. But I must wait. I can't reveal every beauty secret yet. We're only in chapter three.

Before I go on to another verse section, I must jump back to verse 23. "*You'll travel safely; you'll never tire nor trip.*" In our vocation, my husband I travel quite a bit. Last fall, I was on the road eight weekends in a row for speaking engagements. That's a lot of traveling. I love it, I really do. Some people don't enjoy it, but I honestly love the thrill of ordering my airplane ginger ale, quickly making airport connections, driving rental cars, checking into hotels, and even hotel breakfasts. I'm a roadie at heart. I'm a 'nester' in my home, but just as comfortable in the hustle and bustle of road life.

The promise of traveling safely without tiring is incredibly appealing. Yes, please is my response to that thought. Although travel is personally stimulating, it is tiring. How great would it be to still be fully energized after a day of layovers and sitting in the middle seat? My favorite seat is the window seat. I love looking out over the earth, plus you have the side of the plane to lean your head against so you can rest 'without tiring.' See, I so win the aisle vs. window seat battle!

This is just the beginning, my friends. Hopefully this is piquing your interest. Let's do a review. So far, in just four verses, you have the ability to attain fitness, attractiveness, safe non-tiring travels, take afternoon naps without a worry, and enjoy a good night's sleep. Not too shabby.

IF YOU'RE HAPPY AND YOU KNOW IT
(a half chapter)

I know it's not traditional to have a 1/2 chapter in a book. I'm going to break the rules a bit with this, even if I'm walking on the edge! I just wanted a mini chapter to chat how the happiness factor relates to health and beauty. Not too long ago on Facebook, I took a mini poll of all my friends. "What is your #1 beauty tip?" I asked. I had a few responses about particular beauty products, but I also received an overwhelming amount of the same answer. Being happy.

I felt fairly justified in my answer to my newest best friend at The Catfish Hole when asked what my secret to looking young was, and I replied 'I'm happy.' Seems lots of people feel that happiness is a major element in being beautiful. (I have such smart friends.)

I decided to do some of my own research on the subject of happiness and how it relates to our health and physical beauty. Seems my Facebook friends and I are right! My research revealed that there are some amazing benefits to being happy.

I'm sure you've probably heard the term that happiness is a choice. We choose to be happy. Well, we do. It's the glass half full of half empty outlook for life.

We choose how we react in life. We choose every single morning if we are going to walk through our day happy or angry. That single choice affects everyone else we come in contact with that day as well as ourselves.

There are so many studies that have proven that being happy is so beneficial to our well-being as well as our facial beauty. Did you know that in studies scientists have found that being happy can add a minimum of seven years to your life? Seven freebie years to enjoy life from having a positive attitude and smiling. I like that result!

Happy people also have stronger immune systems and lower blood pressure. Don't believe me? Look up all the studies. I'm just condensing the facts I discovered in my research. There are innumerable research findings to prove this is true. Smiling, being positive, laughing, and looking at life with an up-beat view will add years to your life and make you healthier and physically stronger. I'm smiling as I'm writing this, and I think I may have just added a good three days to my life! See, it's easy.

Now anger, on the other hand has unbelievable negative effects to your body. I'm sure most of us are aware how anger affects us emotionally and spiritually, but the physical side effects are staggering.

Research has shown that no matter how much you eat or exercise correctly, you are putting yourself at risk if you do not control your anger. Anger causes a widespread effect on the body. When a person becomes angry, they may experience muscle tension, grinding of the teeth and teeth clenching, ringing in the ears, higher blood pressure, chest pains, excessive sweating, chills, severe headaches or migraines.

Chronic anger is even worse. Seriously, you don't want to exist in a state of anger. Would you like to know the possible side effects? Peptic ulcers, constipation, diarrhea, intestinal cramping, chronic ingestion, heart attacks, strokes, kidney problems, obesity, and frequent colds. The list actually goes on and on. Medical experts have also found that the heart muscle is also affected by anger, and that anger can actually reduce the heart's ability to properly pump blood. Reverse all the negative effects of anger, and you have what a happy person can experience health-wise!

I gotta do it. I have to add a few more negatives with anger. Prolonged anger can also affect your skin! People who hold in their anger may also have skin diseases such as rashes, hives, warts, eczema, and even acne. Unreal, huh!

Unbelievably in research, when people have learned to release their anger, their skin disorders dramatically improve.

I think that's amazing. The Bible tells us to forgive. There is so much anger found in unforgiveness. Jesus teaches us to forgive time after time. God created our physical bodies, and our spiritual selves. He desires us to walk whole both physically and spiritually. He knows that it's all interrelated. What a beautiful benefit of forgiveness—health and beautiful skin. Isn't this great news?

So how does the happiness factor make you prettier? Have you ever taken a good look at angry people? Seriously. I can tell people that aren't happy just by their faces, and the lines on their skin. They look worn from years of scowling. There are different wrinkles from smiling vs. frowning.

Of course, there are many factors to obtaining wrinkles, but from my own personal experience, a wrinkled face from years of joy and laughter is so much more beautiful than a wrinkled face from anger.

Choose to look at life every day with optimism, joy and happiness. It is a daily choice, but the rewards are so great. You will walk healthier and look better, plus, life is so much more enjoyable when you're happy. Those around you will be thankful for your joyful happy spirit, too.

There. My 1/2 chapter is done. Short, sweet, and to the point.

AVON CALLING

I became an Avon Lady at the end of my junior year of high school. Ever since Avon made those miniature lipsticks, I was fascinated with the make-up industry, and especially a company that would deliver beauty products right to your front door. I loved the miniature lipstick samples, and frankly any beauty product that came in a mini size. Don't even get me started on mini fragrance samples. I have a slight addiction problem when it comes to those delightful take-anywhere-try-the-newest-fragrance delights. What's not to love? They're free. They're cute. You smell wonderful.

I became the Avon Lady for our neighborhood (my territory!), and at my high school. That was 1983. Gulp. Sounds so long ago. I was a newbie to the whole world of cosmetics and skin care. I had so much to learn. Looking back, there weren't actually that many anti- wrinkle creams in the early

80's. Skin care was basically divided into three divisions. Oily, normal, and dry. I learned this valuable information from Avon, and the dozens of Mary Kay parties that I was invited to attend during those years.

I remember doing the blot test on my skin with those special thin paper strips. If there was an oily residue, you had oily skin. A slight bit of residue, you had normal skin. Dry skin would sometimes have little flakes of skin on the paper. Gross, I know. I had normal skin with a minute amount of oil in the T-zone.

Dry skin products were aimed at those aged fifty and up. (OLD people skin care). Even in my teen years, I broke all the rules, and usually ended up buying the dry skin systems. Such the rebel. I figured if the dry skin products were to help prevent wrinkles, why not be preventative, and buy the product for wrinkles before you even started getting wrinkles. It may not be correct, but it made great sense to me at the time.

I was in college when the new Avon firming cream was introduced. I was hooked. I always had more defined smile lines (Those folds that appear on either side of the lips running down from the nose). I guess from smiling a lot? Hereditary? Either way, even in my late teens and early twenties they were showing. In college, my dream was to either be in commercials, sing, or be a TV host. With all three career choices, I would need to have my face looking the best it could. It seemed that firming skin care would have to be a vital part of my skin care regimen for the rest of my life.

When I married my husband Dave, I made two personal promises to myself. I wanted to keep my skin looking as young as I could, and to never have a 'mom belly.' Well, I've worked on my skin. And even though my 'baby' is in his twenties, I am still working on getting rid of that baby weight from him. There is something about being over forty when it comes to the belly issue. It's a challenge. I have come to realize that those tall skinny women so have it made.

I have tried my best to keep my skin looking as young as possible. In the twenty-one years that we have been married, there have been many =it' skin care ingredients. Alpha Hydroxy Acid products, Vitamin C serums, and creams infused with retinol have all been advertised as Fountain of Youth products. If each product had actually been everything it claimed to be, there would never be a need for new products. Everyone's wrinkles would have disappeared, and the creator of that product would be set financially for life.

Unfortunately, people continued to get wrinkles, and companies kept searching for the newest and latest miracle product.

This past October, we were privileged to visit Israel and experience the Holy Land. My husband and I were part of the Worship Team for a ministry that does a lot of international crusades, and we were privileged to have ten amazing days in God's country. I had never been to the Holy Land, and absolutely fell in love with the country of Israel. If you've never been, I highly recommend the trip. What an experience to literally see the Bible come alive. The Sea of Galilee was breathtaking, and Jerusalem was everything you could imagine it to be.

One of my favorite Holy Land destinations was the Dead Sea. Of course, I had heard all the stories that you could float in the water, etc. I imagined that the water would be full of floating salt formations, and that the water itself would be almost chunky with salt. Quite the opposite. The water resembled any other body of water I had ever seen. Just regular plain H2O...or so I thought.

We saw what seemed to be 'locals' laying on the beach covered in Dead Sea mud as we walked down to the water. We only had a limited time at the sea, so I wanted to get right to the water. It looked as if the shallow water extended hundreds of feet, because it appeared that the people were just laying down in the sand of the shallow water.

Then I stepped in further. People told me to lay back in the water, and I did so. Oh my. What an unbelievable experience. Yes, indeed, I was floating on this totally normal looking water.

As I was swimming/floating, I felt my skin. My skin felt as soft as a newborn baby. It was utterly amazing. I kept looking at the mud-covered locals, and thought, *If they are covering themselves with this mud, they must know what they are doing.* Every minute was enjoyable, and it was difficult to drag myself out of that heavenly water, but it was well worth the effort.

While we were there my husband and I both completely slathered ourselves with this Dead Sea mud. Black mud as they call it. All we had to do to get the mud was to dig in the mud/sand bottom of the sea. It was abundant. It was free. It was wonderful.

We grabbed two lounge chairs, put them half in the water, and half on the beach, and dried ourselves out. With the delightful arid breezes flowing, it didn't take too long to dry our caked mud-covered bodies.

The real treat came when we floated back into that amazing water to rinse ourselves off. How can I explain this to you in human words? My skin never felt so amazing. Absolutely glorious. It was upon feeling my skin in such a perfect state that it dawned on me that God cares about our physical skin. God himself had created the world's best spa treatment in His beautiful country of Israel. What a gift! The water and mud He created for us to enjoy.

Now some of you may be thinking, 'God doesn't care about spa/mud treatments.' Well, God didn't have to create that sea, or that mud, or place it in a place where people could enjoy the benefits of both, but he did! For thousands and thousands of years, his people have journeyed down to the sea, and have enjoyed such relaxing beauty treatments. There's something about that whole idea I just love. Nowhere else in the world does this same combination of minerals exist. Only in the Dead Sea. The healing waters and 'black mud' of the Dead Sea are one of a kind. A gift to us, and a reminder to me that God created our skin, but he also created ways for us to take care of it!

I read a great book over ten years ago about the beauty industry. The author, a dermatologist, tested and tried every skin care product available: from the cheapest drug store brands to the most expensive imported creams. I quite enjoyed the read, and it was interesting to see what she thought about many of the products I had used over the years. I learned that no-name and high priced brands generally have the same ingredients. Look on the back...read what's in each product and compare the list of ingredients. You'll be surprised at how much money you can save by buying store brands! I also learned some wrinkle prevention information, too.

There are basically two simple ways of preventing wrinkles: stay out of the sun (or use SPF), and live healthy. Smoking, drinking, eating unhealthy foods, and stress are some of the main contributors to wrinkles on your face. Genetics also have a small role to play. If your mom has aged well, chances are that if you do your part, your skin will age gracefully as well. It's actually quite simple.

I grew up in the 70's and 80's, when SPF was basically used for redheads and extremely fair skinned people who tended to burn extremely easily. The youth of my generation tended to use (ouch) baby oil to tan in the sun.

My brother is darker skinned than I am, and always tanned extremely well in a short period of time. I could tan (more golden than actually brown), but it took me a while to build up color.

When my brother and I were in our early teens, we joined our parents in a cross-country RV trip. The RV had orange shag carpeting, and brown paneled walls. I thought it was the coolest thing ever.

Half way through our adventure, we had a pool day in California. My brother was out for an hour, and already had tan lines. I took this California experience as a quest. A quest to get as dark as, if not darker, than my brother. The challenge was on.

I may have been out in the sun 3-4 hours. I don't quite remember how long. I do know that my brother had already gone back to the RV. I kept checking my bathing suit bottom tan lines, and after four hours, was convinced that I had a competition tan.

About three hours later I started to hurt. I indeed had surpassed my brother in color, but the color was red, not brown. I had the worst case of sunburn poisoning ever. It was horrible. Bubbles started forming all over my body, and my temperature skyrocketed. It was beyond bad.

It was weeks until I started healing, and I remember driving back to New Jersey in the RV, while my skin was in its molting stage. It was fun to see how long a piece of skin I could peel. Gross, I know! I had learned my lesson. It was time to leave the baby oil for make-up removal only.

I never wanted to experience sunburn poisoning again. The moral of the story? Limit your sun exposure and wear sunscreen. Learn this very important lesson from my unfortunate experience.

Reading that book ten years ago, I also learned

another important wrinkle fact. Once they're there, you can't do anything to take them away, except for injections or surgery. I know, a harsh reality. Note that the wording on wrinkle creams usually quote, 'To diminish the appearance of fine lines and wrinkles'. The key word is *appearance*. I don't believe there's a beauty cream that can claim that it actually takes away wrinkles. By moisturizing your face, your skin cells will plump up, and give the appearance that your wrinkles have diminished and been filled in.

It is important to moisturize, stay out of the sun, and use a high numbered SPF with limited amounts of sun exposure. Staying out of the sun is your best preventative medicine for future wrinkles. I'm not done with wrinkles though. Much more to come in future chapters. Wrinkles, wrinkles, wrinkles (Marsha, Marsha, Marsha).

I will admit to trying new skin products that come out in the market. I suppose I will always enjoy trying new skin lines and creams. Every person needs to find a great moisturizer that works for their skin. A moisturizer with SPF for the day (or use a foundation with SPF), and a great moisturizing cream for night time. I have tried so many.

For a while, I was using expensive department store brands until I realized that many of the lesser priced products work just as well. Have fun experimenting and trying samples of lotions and serums. Take a good look at your skin after using a product for a while. If you're not happy with the results, or don't think your skin looks good enough for the price you paid, move on to something different.

My quest for the best looking skin possible has led to me use so many different facial products. Although my head knowledge tells me that there isn't the perfect cure for wrinkles, my heart will still go on with the dream that somewhere in the world, someone will concoct the perfect combination of herbs and long forgotten ingredients to actually, once and for all, create the elixir to make wrinkles disappear for good. A girl can dream, can't she?

AND THE RECORD IS: 969 YEARS

It's amazing to me how long people lived in the Old Testament. Methuselah lived to the age of 969. Unbelievable. According to Bible genealogies, Adam lived to be 930 years old, although we don't know what physical age he was when God created him. That's kind of an interesting thought. Even though Adam was created at age zero, he was not created as a baby; he was fully a man. I wonder how old? Eighteen? Thirty-two? I wonder if God created him at the 'perfect' age, perhaps the way we will look when we are in Heaven?

I believe we were actually created to live forever, and not die. Adam and Eve were allowed to eat of the Tree of Life in Eden. It was never forbidden to eat the fruit of that tree.

"Now the LORD God had planted a garden in the east, in Eden; and there he put the man he had formed. The LORD God made all kinds of trees grow out of the ground—trees that were pleasing to the eye and good for food. In the middle of the garden were the tree of life and the tree of the knowledge of good and evil." Genesis 2: 8-9

"The LORD God took the man and put him in the Garden of Eden to work it and take care of it. And the LORD God commanded the man, "You are free to eat from any tree in the garden; but you must not eat from the tree of the knowledge of good and evil, for when you eat from it you will certainly die." Genesis 2:15-17

Adam and Eve, for however many years they were in the garden before they ate of the Tree of Knowledge of Good and Evil, were able to eat fruit from the Tree of Life. We are never told if they actually did, or if the fruit from that tree was part of their everyday diet. Can you imagine how delicious the fruit found in the Garden of Eden must have been?

I believe God intended and created the human being to live forever, multiply, and co-exist in harmony with him. The Tree of Life (eternal physical life I believe) was given to man to eat freely from. It was only after they ate from the Tree of Knowledge of Good and Evil that they were banned to ever eat from the Tree of Life again.

From reading the passages of scripture in Genesis, we can assume that the perfect plan in Eden would have been to be physically sustained by the fruits of the various trees, and for humans to eat from the garden that God created for them.

And God said, "*Behold, I have given you every plant yielding seed which is upon the face of all the earth, and every tree with seed in its fruit; you shall have them for food.*" Genesis 1:29-30

Everything our bodies needed to live perfectly was contained in that garden. This just fascinates me. If there were seasons, how I would love to know what some of the 'Pre-Fall' vegetables and fruits were. Were there different foods and vegetables than what exist today? Our bodies were created perfectly in a perfect world. The physical way we were created was absolute perfection. God designed our bodies, and He also designed the ultimate healthy living and eating environment.

We weren't created to age. Aging and physical death is a result of sin. Biblical scholars believe that physical aging did not exist before sin entered the world, only after the Fall did man start to physically age. Sad, huh.

Now, we fight the aging process with

everything possible. We fight the aging process, and we are also fighting the effects of sin in our physical bodies: sickness and disease. So much in this world changed after the Fall. Those perfect foods that were freely available were now forbidden.

I do believe, though, that God in his grace still gave Adam and Eve healthy fruits and vegetables for consumption, although they had to toil and labor to produce them. It's Interesting that we were physically created to be vegetarians. Actually vegans! So many who turn to the vegan way of life claim that it has changed them for the better physically. If I didn't love In-n-Out burgers so much, I would consider eating vegan. Well, that and it's slightly inconvenient to make brownies without eggs. But if I had to, I think I could.

The American Dietetic Association notes that "most of mankind for most of human history has lived on vegetarian or near-vegetarian diets." Much of the world still lives that way. Even in most industrialized countries, the love affair with meat is less than a hundred years old. It started with the refrigerator car and the twentieth-century consumer society. But even with the twentieth century, man's body hasn't adapted to eating meat.

The prominent Swedish scientist Karl von Linne

states, "Man's structure, external and internal, compared with that of the other animals, shows that fruit and succulent vegetables constitute his natural food."

I grew up as most Americans did; eating all kinds of meat and processed food. Please don't think that the purpose of this chapter is to turn you into a vegetarian or vegan. I just want to consider how God created our bodies to survive.

We weren't given the OK to eat meat until after the Flood. Biblical scholars roughly determine that between the creation of Adam and The Flood in Noah's day, there were 2000 years. That's a long time for vegetarian-only eating. In those two thousand years, humans also lived for extreme amounts of years. The average lifespan of a human before the flood was 857 years! That's unbelievable! The vegan way of eating is looking better and better the more I write!

Many creationists believe that there was a pre-flood water canopy surrounding the earth, which kept the earth a tropical paradise. Genesis 1:7 states that God created 'the waters above the firmament.' This theory states that the waters above the firmament were a 'vast blanket of invisible water vapor...productive of a marvelous greenhouse effect which maintained mild temperatures from pole to pole, thus preventing air-mass circulation and the resultant rainfall. It would certainly have had the further effect of efficiently filtering harmful radiation from space, markedly reducing the rate of somatic mutations in living cells, and, as a consequence, drastically decreasing the rate of aging and death." (Morris, Henry, Scientific Creationism, 1984, p. 211.)

Even though man was not permitted to live forever physically and abide in the perfectly created Garden of Eden, there were benefits to living in the pre-flood earth. I believe the whole earth changed after the flood. The physical properties changed. The firmament that surrounded the earth and created the greenhouse effect caused vegetation to grow abundantly (even with the curse of 'toiling in the earth'), and the atmosphere was such that humans could live to the average age of 857 years! What a world!

Unfortunately, God was not pleased with how his human creation was turning out. You know the story of Noah and the ark. Then the LORD said, "*My Spirit will not put up with humans for such a long time, for they are only mortal flesh. In the future, their normal lifespan will be no more than 120 years.*" (Genesis 6:3)

Even though Noah lived to be 950 years old, the generations following him drastically declined in lifespan percentages. Although it took twelve generations for man to average the 120 years for a life, no one after Noah lived even near the 900 year age mark. I guess God meant it when he said it, and it happened!

What is interesting to me is that when God declared man would only live to 120, which was a drastic difference, only then did he gave the command that eating meat was allowed. Perhaps meat eating was a variable in the shortened human lifespan?

The current U.S. Life expectancy is 77.5 years. This number takes the current rates of mortality at each age and figures out where the average is. Unfortunately, because of disease, lifestyle and I believe, processed foods, we are living 42.5 years below what our optimum lifespan should be. Think of the great things you could accomplish with an additional 42.5 years to your life!

If Adam and Eve had not sinned and eaten the forbidden fruit, I would never be writing this book. We would never age. We would live forever in perfect condition. Someday we will all have new bodies. Perfect bodies. Ageless bodies.

Until the day that I leave this earth, and attain that heavenly body, I want to live to my optimum. There's no reason why humans shouldn't be living to 120. What should we adjust in our everyday lives to live to our fullest? Beauty is attained when we live at our full potential physically, spiritually, and mentally.

Do I have to give up cotton candy (one of my favorites), brownies (another favorite), steak, chicken, and eggs to live to 120? Possibly. Would it be worth it? It all depends. I want to enjoy my years on this planet. I also desire to be a healthy and beautiful temple for the Holy Spirit. I said it before: my goal is to live to 100. Perhaps 100 is attainable with eating brownies and animal products. If so, I could be satisfied. That would be a good life. But if God impresses upon me to try to make it to the 120 mark, I may have to give up that cotton candy.

You may be asking, "Why include the biblical history of age in a book about beauty?" I know it's not your typical chapter you might find in other books, but it's important to know that God created us to live at a higher life potential than I believe most of us attaining, myself included.

A beautiful person is a person walking fulfilled in every aspect of life. Being all that we can and should be is our gift back to God.

FESTOONED WITH BEAUTY

I've got to jump back into those wonderful hidden secret promises in Proverbs. Of course, if they're in the Bible, they're not really secret...they've been there for thousands of years. It's just that I've never heard anyone teach on them, and they've never stood out as anything special to me until I started my research for beauty tips. Now I will guard these golden nuggets of scripture with my life, and do my best to follow the wise instructions.

"Above all and before all, do this: Get Wisdom! Write this at the top of your list: Get Understanding! Throw your arms around her believe me, you won't regret it; never let her go— she'll make your life glorious. She'll garland your life with grace, she'll festoon your days with

beauty. Dear friend, take my advice; It will add years to your life." Proverbs 4: 7-10

Where to begin? That's the question. That's all so good! I enjoy learning new things. I really do. I don't ever want to stop learning, or come to the place where I think I have learned it all. Albert Einstein wrote the words, "When you stop learning, you start dying." Smart man. I believe just the fact that you're reading this book, and wanting to learn more about taking care of yourself is seeking after wisdom. Wisdom in God's ways, and also wisdom of living our lives to their fullest is the key.

This portion from the book of Proverbs has four promises for seeking after Wisdom and Understanding. The first promise is that Wisdom will make your life glorious. Not too shabby of a promise. I want to live a glorious life!

glo·ri·ous Adjective

1. Having, worthy of, or bringing fame or admiration: "glorious victory". 2. Having a striking beauty or splendor that evokes feelings of delighted admiration.

I enjoy looking up the definitions for words. I think so many times we (myself included) throw out words in our vocabulary that we really don't know the definition of. I, in particular, appreciate the #2 definition of glorious. I would love for every part of my life to have 'striking beauty.' Women pay thousands and thousands of dollars to attain striking beauty. Save the money; just seek after Wisdom.

Now don't get me wrong, I'm not saying you can just sit around seeking after wisdom and 'striking beauty' will suddenly appear. That's like wishing you had a plate full of brownies, and you want them to magically appear on your lap. You have to get up, get all of your ingredients ready, do the physical act of stirring, mixing, and baking them in the oven. Then, after you have done all the work, you can enjoy those delicious chewy on the insides, crunchy on the corners delightfully satisfying treats. (And now all I want is one of them...) Brownies are a weakness of mine; can you tell?

I feel that seeking after wisdom, and following the 'secrets' you have found, and then applying what you have learned is the key here. This book is about beauty: inside as well as outside. If you learned that using a moisturizer with SPF would prevent further wrinkles and didn't apply that wisdom to your life, then you would be throwing out that new found wisdom, and the 'glorious' benefits mentioned in this portion of Proverbs.

Seek after Wisdom, apply the wisdom that you have learned, and then you will reap the benefits. Great benefits by the way, too!

I understand that the Wisdom mentioned in Proverbs 4:7-10 is seeking after God's ways, and his 'statutes.' Well, he made our skin, and he knows the effects of skin damage, too! I really don't mean to question God's ways here, but I know that God desires us to live full and healthy lives. Over exposure to the sun leads to skin damage, and possible skin cancer. I would believe that having skin cancer is not something in God's perfect plan for our lives.

So, if you came across the information that skin cancer is preventable, found out that simply not over exposing your skin to the sun and using SPF could prevent that damage, wouldn't it be wise for you to take that wisdom, and do everything possible in prevention?

"She'll garland your life with grace, she'll festoon your days with beauty.' Garland and festoon aren't every day common vernacular. We usually use the word garland once a year: at Christmas. Garland, in the form that we are used to seeing, is typically a long strand of fake pine. I love to garland our staircase with garland. Did you notice that I just used garland as a verb and a noun? Elementary school teachers reading this book will be proud of me, thank you very much.

The official definition is below:

gar·land Verb: Adorn or crown with a garland. Noun: A wreath of flowers and leaves, worn on the head or hung as a decoration.

So according to the verse, grace (a state of sanctification/to make holy, purify) will be upon your head in the form of a crown of purity and holiness. I love that. I'm not much of a hat person, but I'd surely take a crown of holiness. That's the inner beauty that shines out through us.

Solomon also tells us that Wisdom will 'festoon your days with beauty'. Thanks goodness for dictionary access on the internet. I can quickly look up these unfamiliar words. I honestly don't think I've ever had the word festoon come out of my mouth.

fes·toon

Noun: A chain or garland of flowers, leaves, or ribbons, hung in a curve as a decoration. Verb: Adorn (a place) with chains, garlands, or other decorations: "the room was festooned with balloons."

Now that I know what the word means, I think I may have to just throw it around a bit. People will think I'm so much smarter than I really am. This will be fun.

Apparently festoon and garland are closely related words, almost interchangeable. I like the thought of having my days decorated with beauty for simply seeking after Wisdom. See, I told you there were some amazing beauty secrets hidden in these scriptures!

The best promise out of this passage has to be the last phrase, "Dear friend, take my advice; it will add years to your life."

Americans are quite obsessed with living longer, and rightly so. The more we're on this earth, the more of an impact we can make, and the more lives we can touch. I want to live a full life. There are books and books on living longer. Yet, within one simple passage of scripture, we just read how to attain a long life! That answer has been sitting in our Bible for thousands of years! Follow Solomon's words and wisdom in Proverbs, and a long life is yours. Simple, huh?

Here are some more:

"The ways of right-living people glow with light; the longer they live, the brighter they shine". Proverbs 4: 18

Now if that isn't an encouraging verse, I don't know what is! The average American believes that growing older is a downhill road. You start to shrink (literally), lose muscle and bone mass, wrinkle, shrivel and then die.

This Proverbs verse gives hope! Be a right-living person, and you will glow with light, and as you grow older, you will shine brighter and brighter. Now after reading that, would you seriously consider being a wrong-living person?

Gain all the knowledge and wisdom you can. Never stop learning. Abraham Lincoln said, "I don't think much of a man who is not wiser today than he was yesterday." The verses mentioned in this chapter are rich. Rich with wisdom, and rich with hope. We don't have to decline as we age. We can grow more beautiful, glow, shine, and live long lives. I'm encouraged just writing this. What hope! What delicious beauty and longevity secrets.

LOOKIN' GOOD

Outward physical beauty.

At the writing of this book there are currently 17,889 paperback books available on beauty! If there wasn't a demand, there wouldn't be that many books. That's a staggering amount of books written for women across the world desiring to look their best physically.

I know there's a school of thought that to be concerned with your physical appearance is vanity. I have been fascinated with the beauty industry ever since my early teen years and I don't consider myself to be a non-spiritual vain person. I thrive daily to be all that God desires me to be, but I also want to look my physical best. I believe both are possible.

I love beauty products. I love the way they make my skin feel. I enjoy trying new products when they come on the market. I search out the latest and best skin care lines. I experiment. I sample. I could spend the afternoon at beauty counters in stores trying lotions and serums, and be completely satisfied. I love gift-with-purchase bags that contain trial size skin care products. That's just the kind of girl I am!

I gotta say, I think my husband is glad I'm that kind of girl, too. I am so thankful that my hubby loves me when I look plain and simple. To be honest, that's roughly five days out of the week. But, when the make-up is applied (in a tasteful fashion, of course) he looks at me with a twinkle in his eye. I like that. After twenty-one years of marriage, to still get a twinkle is saying something.

He likes when I put an effort forth to look my best. Now there's a freebie marital relationship tip, girls. Just threw that in. My husband will often tell me, "Thank you for taking the time to look your best."

Before I got married, I happened across the book, *His Needs, Her Needs: Building An Affair-Proof Marriage* written by Willard E. Harley, Jr. It's one of the best marital books written, I believe. The book has sold over a million copies. Dr. Harley is a marriage therapist, and defines the top five needs of both men and women in a marriage.

The top five for men are: sexual fulfillment,

recreational companionship, an attractive spouse, domestic support, and admiration. Granted, sexual fulfillment placed higher than an attractive spouse, but really, that shouldn't come as a huge surprise. The possible surprise here is that out of all the things in the world that a man could desire in a marital relationship, having a spouse that is attractive is #3!

A man needs a wife who looks good to him. Dr. Harley states that in sexual relationships most men find it nearly impossible to appreciate a woman for her inner qualities alone — there must be more. A man's need for physical attractiveness in a mate is profound.

"A man with a need for an attractive spouse feels good whenever he looks at his attractive wife. In fact, that is what emotional needs are all about. When one of his emotional needs is met he feels fulfilled, and when it's not met, he feels frustrated. It may sound immature or superficial, but I've found that most men have a need for an attractive wife. They do not appreciate a woman for her inner qualities alone. They appreciate the way she looks." Dr. Willard E. Harley, Jr.

Note that those words are written by a marriage therapist, and not someone that sells cosmetics. Dr. Harley has been a well-respected therapist for decades who has dealt with thousands of men and women across the country. I, for one, want to have the best non-affair marriage possible. If having an attractive spouse is #3 in a list of ways to keep your husband satisfied in a marriage, then I want to do as much as I possibly can to keep him fulfilled.

Now don't think I'm suggesting make-up 24/7, and to never let your husband see you without being made up. That would be craziness. Really. I am suggesting though, putting forth an effort to learn to look your best.

Find out what kind of make-up your husband prefers. Is he a 'just lip gloss' kind of guy, or does he appreciate a face with full mascara, eye shadow, blush, and lipstick applications? You'll know you've hit the bull's-eye when he mentions how great you look.

Some of you may feel that your husband doesn't care what you look like. Well, do you care what he looks like? Do you remember those nervous butterflies you felt when you were just starting to date, and you'd see him walk around the corner? Yes, you were attracted to his soul, but honestly, you were also attracted by what you saw. I, for one, don't want my husband to just 'let it go.' I married him for all of his characteristics, and his good looks and physique were included in those characteristics.

Age happens, additional pounds happen, hair loss happens, but as long as my husband does his best to look his best, I am satisfied. Books and books have been written about the power of physical attraction. It's real.

I didn't know anything about my future husband's personality when I initially met him, but I did know that I was overwhelmingly attracted to his physical appearance. He was 100% my type physically. Thank goodness he had the personality and spiritually to match those good looks!

I'm sure Dave had his first impressions of me, too. Thank goodness I was skinnier back then! Don't get me wrong, the outward appearance isn't everything. I would be way off course in life if I believed that, but outward appearance does count.

When we were dating, I'd spend extra time getting ready to look my best. I wanted to look pretty for him. Unfortunately, so many married women don't think they have to be 'looking pretty' for their husbands anymore. They got the ring, now they can relax and not worry about how they look anymore.

The key, especially in marriage, is not to totally let ourselves go. We need to throw out the theory that "Well, now that I got him to marry me, it doesn't really matter how I look." It's my desire to do my best to keep myself the best I can be for my husband. I certainly don't live in fear that if I gain a few pounds, and don't wear make-up every day that my husband is going to leave me.

I don't live in a fairytale world where physical perfection is the standard. Trust me. I have gained weight since we were married, and I often wear sweats and baseball caps during the day. But I do know how to (as my husband says) 'clean up.'

I love it when, after a day in sweats, I go get ready, and he smiles and says, "Boy, you sure do clean up well" with a twinkle in his eye. I see that cleaning up as a little gift from me to him.

If you're not married yet, take this advice: look your best. Fix up. Men are attracted to women on a physical level. Just the way it is. I have met so many single women that just don't understand why they're not married.

Can I be honest here? Some of these gals have done nothing to make themselves look good. You don't have to slather the blush and lipstick to look good, but put some kind of effort forth. Get your hair styled. Have your nails done. Splurge on some new outfits. (I'm the thriftiest shopper around. You can find great clothes on a tight budget). Cut back on desserts. A little eye make-up goes a long way. Accenting your face with some color will make you stand out. It's the 'thrill of the hunt' for men. Putting forth effort to look your best will get results. You'll start to turn the heads of those single men! It's worth it, girls!

Dave loves me fancy or in gym attire, but I make it a point to still put forth the effort to fix up, and look my best. A supermodel I will never be. I just don't have that genetic DNA (sorry birth mom and dad, but it's true). Sometimes I'll see a tall slender woman, and say to my husband, "Sorry I don't have those genes", and I'm fortunate enough to hear the response, "Oh stop, you're perfect just the way you are." I love that man of mine.

There is a three-second theory. Within the first three seconds of meeting someone new, based on their physical appearance, you have your first impressions already made. That's just our nature. It happens. This three-second theory not only relates to our spouses, but to everyone we come in contact with. Some may say that first impressions aren't important. I disagree.

When I go to speak somewhere new, especially to a group of women, I know that they are checking me out. We women are good at checking each other out. We make a justified glance from the top of their hair to the shoes they are wearing within seconds. Instantly we decide if we like them or not. If the 'new one' will be someone we can relate to, or if we are from totally different worlds. Hate to say it, but the classy/non-classy judgment is also made. Come on, now, get real with me. We all do it. First impressions can be changed, but nonetheless, we make them. You would have a totally different first impression of me if you met me right now (typing in my sweats with messy hair and no make-up) than you would if you saw me Sunday morning singing up on the platform.

When going into a new environment and meeting new people, I put forth the effort to present the best me that I can. Along with a smile and a friendly handshake or hug, I want to represent a positive and outgoing first impression.

Appropriate dress, hair fixed, fragrance, make-up, and some accessories are my 'staples.' I'm a wife, mother, speaker, singer, and most importantly a follower of Christ. I want my outward appearance to match my inward qualities, and to represent to the best of my ability who I am on the inside by what I present on the outside.

Let's consider the three-second impression. That's not a lot of time. Beauty: learning tools to represent your inner beauty on your outward canvas. A challenge, but a challenge with rewards and satisfaction. May I mirror on the outward the joy and love on the inside, and that my first three seconds of impression time impress someone enough that they will take the time to get to know who I really am.

SMOOTHIES AND SIT-UPS

"*Dear friend, listen well to my words; tune your ears to my voice. Keep my message in plain view at all times. Concentrate! Learn it by heart! Those who discover these words really live; body and soul they're bursting with health.*" Proverbs 4:20-22

When I was in college, the only 'workout equipment' the gym had were copper colored exercise bikes with plastic knobs to adjust the tension on the front wheel. Those bikes, a track, and a stinky sweat-filled room filled with jocks and free weights were my options. Not much incentive to workout.

When Dave and I started dating, I joined a Bally Health Club. It cost about $200+ to join, and then

$35 a month. The best part of Bally in 1989 was that there were free tanning beds. Oh, I used those beds! Sometimes I'd tan at one club in the morning and another in the evening. I was delightfully tan and in great shape.

I am not a morning person, but the only time during the day that I could meet my then boyfriend, was to workout at 6 a.m. I still can't believe I went to the gym at 6 a.m.! The crazy things you will do when you're in love. My word.

Even though my main incentive to join the gym was for free tanning and to meet my boyfriend, I did gain the additional benefit of getting in great shape. I became a master on the stair step machine, thank you very much. The stair step machine was the newest popular machine back then. The elliptical wasn't even invented yet. I remember doing an hour straight each time. Oh yeh, I looked good.

My life back then consisted of the gym, eating TCBY frozen yogurt, and Lean Cuisine frozen dinners. I was skinny, fairly healthy, and I felt great. 1989 was the first year of being a health club member, and the start of seeing the difference having a regular workout schedule can make. I was 24 years old. I saw faster results than now, at 48. Regardless, the 'get-in-shape bug' had bitten me.

The beauty benefits of getting in shape are

endless. Do you want a few reasons for you to add exercise to your daily regimen? Then consider the benefits that exercise has on the skin. There are a number of ways in which you can benefit from exercise.

Sure, you can lose a few pounds. But, did you know that your skin can actually benefit from exercise as well? This is very true and you can reap the rewards right away too. Exercise is something that the body needs, no matter what.

Here are some ways in which it can help your skin to look amazing and to glow without the help of any chemicals and treatments.

• Reduces your acne. Believe it or not, you can reduce the amount of acne that you have on your body, especially your face. Exercise will get the body moving and will therefore create sweat. Think sweat is a bad thing? It can help to keep your pores cleaned out and help remove harmful chemicals that are stored deep in them. Also, it can help by mediating the testosterone hormones in the skin, which cause acne in the first place.

• Increased circulation. If you get in a regular workout in, you are likely to increase the circulation in your body. This will promote the increased delivery of nutrients to the skin cells.

Toxins are also on the out. By increasing circulation of the blood in your body, you will be adding quite a benefiting factor to your skin. It can also help in making collagen and keep the wrinkles at bay.

• De-stressing you. By exercising, your body can help you to be less stressed. There are plenty of ways in which this is beneficial to your body and overall health. The skin is no different. Being less stressed will encourage more of a natural glow to your skin.

Proverbs 4:20-22 tells us that if you once again follow the words of Solomon your body and soul will burst with health. Of course, you need to read the words, follow the advice, and apply it to your everyday life. It needs to become routine.

The pursuit of health drives a majority of Americans, and people across the world. Books, diets, whole grocery store chains, TV shows, and infomercials are centered on the goal of living healthy lives. That goal drives people to spend millions of their hard earned dollars. The answers to what they are searching for I will give you.

Really! They're sitting in Proverbs. Now, I don't have the miracle cure for health problems, but I believe the verses I will share contain preventative wisdom, and insight regarding how to live well, and healthy.

We already read in Proverbs 3:24 that seeking after Wisdom and Common Sense gives you the result of enjoying a good night's sleep. This is one of the best health tips. Sleep, sleep, sleep. We are being created on a life cycle dependent upon sleep and proper rest. Getting the proper amount of sleep can help you lose weight.

Researchers have found that people who sleep less than 7 hours a night are more likely to be overweight and obese. It is thought that the lack of sleep impacts the balance of hormones in the body that affect appetite. The hormones ghrelin and leptin, important for the regulation of appetite, have been found to be disrupted by lack of sleep. Researchers at the University of Chicago found that dieters who were well rested lost more fat, 56% of their weight loss, than those who were sleep deprived, who lost more muscle mass.

Getting enough sleep also helps you reduce stress. When your body is sleep deficient, it goes into a state of stress. The body's functions are put on high alert which causes an increase in blood pressure and production of stress hormones. Higher blood pressure increases your risk for heart attacks and strokes. The stress hormones also, unfortunately, make it harder for you to sleep.

Do you have problems with inflammation? Getting enough sleep will *also* help you with that. Inflammation is linked to heart disease, stroke, diabetes, arthritis and premature aging. Research indicates that people who get less sleep—six or fewer hours a night—have higher blood levels of inflammatory proteins than those who get more.

A 2010 study found that C-reactive protein, which is associated with heart attack risk, was higher in people who got six or fewer hours of sleep a night. People who have sleep apnea or insomnia can have an improvement in blood pressure and inflammation with treatment of the sleep disorders.

Want to live longer? Yep. Also related to sleep! Too much or too little sleep is associated with a shorter lifespan, although it's not clear if it's a cause or effect. (Illnesses may affect sleep patterns too.)

In a 2010 study of women ages 50 to 79, more deaths occurred in women who got less than five hours of sleep per night. "Sleep also affects quality of life. Many things that we take for granted are affected by sleep," says Raymonde Jean, MD, director of sleep medicine and associate director of critical care at St. Luke's-Roosevelt Hospital Center in New York City. "If you sleep better, you can certainly live better. It's pretty clear."

And last but not least at all, it makes you look more beautiful! While you sleep your body produces more protein, allowing cells to repair damage – including those harmed from ultraviolet rays (sun damage) and pollution. Getting your 8 hours can also result in more human growth hormone production (HGH). HGH works to retain skin elasticity, making you less likely to wrinkle.

Sleep is equally as important as diet and exercise to a healthy body; and a healthy body is a beautiful body. Sleeping about 8 hours a night reduces puffy, red eyes, dark under-eye circles and pale or washed- out complexions. Furthermore, new research has shown that those who do get enough sleep (from 7-9 hours a night) are more likely to lose weight and keep it off. This is because sleep reduces the stress hormone cortisol that controls our appetite, raises blood sugar levels and promotes fat to be stored on our abdomen.

There. Is that enough information to keep you in that bed of yours for at least 7 1/2 hours a night? There are more benefits to list, but I believe you can see the importance of sleep. I, for one, love sleeping. Some people have told me they can easily survive on 4 hours of sleep a night. I need a good eight hours, and have no problem going a little longer. There are also incredible creativity benefits to longer sleep. I'll take all the creative help I can get!

Now I realize that 8-10 hours of sleep a night being beneficial to your health and beauty isn't necessarily a brand new 'secret.' But I'll almost bet you didn't realize that it was a bonus benefit of following after God's wisdom.

It's kind of like an algebraic equation. A=B, B=C, therefore A=C. The transitive property. I just looked it up to be sure. If Seeking after God's wisdom=A good night's sleep, and A good night's sleep=Health and beauty benefits, therefore Seeking after God's wisdom=Health and beauty benefits.

Some math teacher somewhere should be very proud of me at this very moment for applying an algebraic equation to represent a non-mathematical situation.

"Body and soul they are bursting with health" (Proverbs 4:22). I love the thought of bursting with health. I believe we were put on this earth to burst with health and not to walk defeated in mind and body. If proper sleep will contribute to my optimum health (and also provide additional beauty bonuses), then hand me my pillow. It's nap time! Actually I can't nap quite yet. I want to finish writing this chapter. I've got some more golden nuggets to share with you.

"Oh listen dear child—become wise; point your

life in the right direction. Don't drink too much wine and get drunk; don't eat too much food and get fat. Drunks and gluttons will end up on skid row, in a stupor and dressed in rage." Proverbs 23:20-21.

Where to begin with this section? This one is loaded. Whew. My liberal friends will love this, my ultra- conservatives won't be happy, but this is in the Bible. "Don't drink too much wine." It's pretty obvious that this verse is telling us that it's not a sin or wrong to drink wine. This is scripture here, friends. Remember, Jesus' first miracle was to turn water into wine.

Wine is not bad. It's actually quite good for you. Wine contains flavonoids and tannins which are components shown to prevent cardiovascular disease, strokes, liver disease, and diabetes. Study after study (I won't bore you with citing them all) in scientific environments prove how beneficial 1-2 glasses of wine a day can be.

The American Heart Association does back the Biblical evidence that excessive drinking of wine can cause the opposite. The risk of cardiovascular disease, strokes, and heart attacks are actually increased with the abuse of wine consumption. The Bible. It will always prove itself true.

Now, before some of you get all uptight with the thought that I'm promoting alcohol, relax. Even though wine would be quite beneficial to my health, I actually don't like the taste of it. I'm not against it, it just doesn't appeal to my taste buds. Liberal Christian friends will have pity on me, and my conservatives are now breathing a sigh of relief. All is good.

Food. Excessive food consumption. I could write a whole book on this topic alone. Many people have. It amuses me how many will point a finger and condemn those who might enjoy a glass of red wine, yet they themselves have no problem gorging themselves at an all-you-can-eat buffet. Ouch. Truth. Overindulgence with both wine and food is wrong, and unhealthy. I'm quoting Solomon here. Remember: God made him the wisest man to have ever lived.

Telling you that obesity is an out of control disease would be no new news. We hear and read about it every day. It just slightly amuses me that in the church especially, it's not thought of as a problem, and it's accepted. This book is on beauty secrets and living healthy lives.

Portion control and what you eat is as important as any beauty tip available. What you put in your mouth, and the quantity you put in your mouth affects your mind, spirit, and your physical body. We are the temple of the Holy Spirit. It is our responsibility to do our utmost to make sure our 'temple' is in its optimum condition.

You want a beauty secret? Follow Solomon's advice 'Don't get fat.' It's simple. Don't gorge yourself. Eat healthy options. Be wise about what you put in your mouth. There's a simple rule for eating proper amounts for our bodies. This is simple. This will hopefully be easy for you to remember. It has stuck with me. When it comes to meal sizes, look at your hand. The palm of your hand is an appropriate measuring tool for meat portion.

Your thumb represents an ounce of cheese that is allotted. One fist is a portion of pasta/rice. Two fists are the size allowed for greens/vegetables. Isn't that easy!

Next time you're in the buffet line, take a looksee at your hand, and eat moderately. You'll be thankful, and much healthier!

You can read the consequences of where 'drunks and gluttons' end up. It's not a happy ending situation. Moderation is the key word yet again in this passage. Don't drink too much, and don't overeat. Overdoing either is a straight shot to an unhealthy lifestyle, and 'Skid Row.'

I quite enjoy the present street I live on. I don't want to end up on Skid Row. I don't want you to end up there, either. Moderation and wisdom. Four easy steps to beauty and a healthy life: Exercise, sleep, don't over indulge in wine, and don't overeat. If you follow just these four lifestyle patterns, I can almost guarantee you 'A life bursting with health.' When you're healthy on the inside, it shines on the outside. Isn't that what we all really want?

THOSE LAST TEN POUNDS...

This is what I call fun chapter time. I want to basically overload you with some great diet secrets. Just a bunch of tips. Some may be repeats you've heard before, but if there's only one new tip that you've never heard that aids you in looking and feeling your best, then this will be a chapter worth reading.

Actually, as I'm typing this, I'm changing my mind. I don't want to give you diet secrets. I don't want to talk about diets in the form of a quick fix to losing weight, rather the lifestyle of eating right.

For most of my adult married life, I have tried various diets. Do you remember the Cabbage Soup Diet? A friend of ours lost a bunch of weight following it, so we got pretty excited; bought all the ingredients we needed, and started. I cooked the cabbage soup on the first day and ate it. It actually surprised us that it was quite yummy.

The second day we heated up the big batch, and consumed our quantities. It was OK. Not as tasty as on the first day. By the third day of heating up that stuff, I could barely stomach the soggy cabbage leaves. Ugh. I guess I'm just not made for boring food diets.

I am always hoping that the next diet plan will provide that magic formula to really getting weight off, and getting back to the number on the scale that I want to see again. A few years ago I did use a diet that worked for a while. We ate Special K cereal, and ate Light Progresso soups. The soups (for a huge can) range from 100 to 160 calories. I got that diet from a friend that had lost 30 pounds in two months. I calculated that I dropped around 18 pounds, which is amazing. It really did work.

The only thing is that now I can't even think of eating more of that soup. I could, and it would probably work again, but it gags me slightly, because I consumed so much of it last year that I can't think about consuming it again in those quantities.

So, do crash diets work? Yup. Can you remain on them? Some of you could. Honestly, if I knew that to remain healthy or to kick a disease, I'd have to eat only Light Progresso soups, I could totally do it. I might gag a bit, but in order to live, it would be possible. The question is, do I want to eat those soups on a regular basis? No. I love variety. I so enjoy baking and cooking.

With so many strict crash diets in the marketplace, so many can't be maintained. If they could, there wouldn't be a need for any more 'new breaking' diets. Everyone that wanted to lose weight would just be able to follow that one diet, and the world would be a happy skinny place.

I have gained twenty pounds since I married Dave twenty-five years ago. I am not obese. I am not overly fat. I've heard that the average woman gains 1 pound per year she is married. I am smack dab average. The only thing is I don't want to continue being average. No more pounds, please. I would love to be back to my marriage weight, though.

The problem is, I don't want to just limit myself to eating certain soups, or cutting out bread and carbs (which I just happen to love). That brings me to decision time. Am I willing to stop eating foods that I enjoy to get back to my desired weight, or am I satisfied being twenty pounds over my goal weight, but to still have the freedom to eat what I want? The last option has been winning, but with moderation.

The other day at the gym, I was thinking, *I eat properly, I go to the gym, and still I am staying at this same weight. Perhaps I should just be satisfied where I am.* Then I went home, and tried on the bathing suit I bought last season for this summer. Wrong, wrong, wrong. Guess I never want to be just satisfied.

Age and DNA are catching up. I really have noticed a metabolism difference since hitting forty. The other factor is that I don't have tall super skinny people in my hereditary line. My 'people' just aren't created to be Sports Illustrated Supermodels. I wish they were, but there's absolutely nothing I can do about that now.

I know that I can maintain my current weight by exercising on a fairly regular basis, and by eating moderate portions of food. We even bought the smaller sized paper plates (there's a bonus weight loss tip) to eat on. Don't be horrified. The glass plates only come out when we have company. Paper plates are the standard in my house. Plus, we really do eat less because the plate looks full. On a full sized glass plate, our portions would look small. I'll take any trick I can get!

So, here are some of those tips and tricks I promised. Some of you may have heard about for years, some may be new. Take them or leave them: it's all up to you. I just want to be the messenger.

Some may sound simple, but every little bit helps. I want you to be the best *you* you can be. Isn't that what we all really want anyway? Be the person God created us to be, take the genetic DNA He created us with, and live at our optimum level. Not diet at our optimum, but live. I can't live on a diet of no carbohydrates. For a short time, yes, but I need to find an eating plan that I can maintain for life.

OK, enough chatting. You want some tips to help you? Here you go:

Stop Drinking Soda

I know you may not see this as a new tip. But, I can't believe how many people are still drinking their empty calories. Want some crazy facts about soda? If you were to consume two glasses of soda a day (and that's not a lot for some), you'll gain a pound a week from them. That's 52 POUNDS in a YEAR from drinking sodas ALONE! That's horrible!

I love root beer. It is my soda of choice. I have limited myself to having root beer usually only if we are having pizza, and on very rare occasions. I don't know what it is, but there is just something about the way pizza and root beer go together. I need to also add, that I'll only order root beer with pizza if we are in a restaurant. 99% of the time that we eat out, I (as well as my whole family) order ice water with lemon slices. There are two benefits to ordering ice water. It's FREE, and it's so much healthier.

It's all your decision. I am not going to force you to give up drinking soda. I'm not. I just want you to be informed that two a day for a year could put 52 extra pounds of fat on your body. That's a staggering number.

Even diet sodas aren't that great for you. A few years ago, I thought I would go .all diet drinks. In our home. Then I read about the effects of aspartame. That knowledge ruined my diet drink decision. There are 92 different negative health side effects of the artificial sweetener. Aspartame dissolves into solution and can therefore travel throughout the body and deposit within any tissue. The body digests aspartame unlike saccharin, which does not break down within humans.

What does that mean? I'll tell you. Here are ways that aspartame (found in almost ALL diet/sugar-free drinks) will affect your health:

-Eye blindness in one or both eyes decreased vision and/or other eye problems such as: blurring, bright flashes, squiggly lines, tunnel vision, decreased night vision pain in one or both eyes decreased tears trouble with contact lenses bulging eyes.

-Ear tinnitus, ringing or buzzing sound severe intolerance of noise marked hearing impairment.

-Neurologic epileptic seizures, headaches, migraines and (some severe) dizziness, unsteadiness, both confusion, memory loss, both severe drowsiness and sleepiness paresthesia or numbness of the limbs severe slurring of speech.

-Severe hyperactivity and restless legs atypical facial pain severe tremors.

-Psychological/Psychiatric severe depression irritability aggression.

-Anxiety personality changes insomnia phobias.

-Chest palpitations, tachycardia shortness of breath recent high blood pressure.

-Gastrointestinal nausea diarrhea, sometimes with blood in stools abdominal pain. Pain when swallowing.

-Skin and Allergies itching without a rash lip and mouth reactions hives aggravated respiratory allergies such as asthma.

-Endocrine and Metabolic loss of control of diabetes menstrual changes marked thinning or loss of hair marked weight loss.

-Gradual weight gain aggravated low blood sugar (hypoglycemia) severe PMS.

-Other frequency of voiding and burning during urination excessive thirst, fluid retention, leg swelling, and bloating increased susceptibility to infection.

-Death, irreversible brain damage birth defects, including mental retardation, peptic ulcers aspartame addiction and increased craving for sweets hyperactivity in children severe depression aggressive behavior suicidal tendencies.

-Aspartame may trigger, mimic, or cause the following illnesses: Chronic Fatigue Syndrome Epstein-Barr Post-Polio Syndrome.

-Lyme Disease Grave's Disease Meniere's Disease Alzheimer's Disease ALS.

-Epilepsy Multiple Sclerosis (MS) EMS

-Hypothyroidism

-Mercury sensitivity from Amalgam fillings

-Fibromyalgia

-Lupus Non-Hodgkin's Lymphoma Attention Deficit Disorder (ADD).

I know! It's almost as if I just sent you through shock treatment at a psychiatric hospital! If you never knew all of that information, you now do. You are welcome.

It's unbelievably shocking isn't it? After I found out all of those side effects, I started looking at 'diet' product labels. Aspartame is in nearly every product. Now wonder there are so many illnesses as of late! Look what we're doing to ourselves!

If the only reason you bought this book was to have the information I just gave you, then it is all worth it. Stay safe. Stay healthy.

I know processed white sugar has received a bad rap, but in comparison, bring on the natural white stuff! Again, as with everything, moderation is the key word. White sugar is not the best for our bodies, but it sure won't affect you the way aspartame will. Now you have the knowledge. Check those labels.

Splenda and now stevia have shown to be better options when going sugar-free. Recent reports have come out with some negatives against Splenda, but they aren't nearly as bad as aspartame.

Stevia, one of the newest alternatives, is 100% natural, and comes from the Stevia rebaudiana plant. Japan has been using these sweet leaves for decades. They're always so ahead of us. I say go natural. It's always better. Stevia is available at Walmart and other grocery stores. Check it out. You can always make your sweet tea and Kool-Aid drinks with it. The decision is yours.

Drink ICE Water

Drinking water for your health is not new news. The benefits are staggering. Drinking water helps to prevent so many disorders. Hydration helps the body naturally replenish its supply of the neurotransmitter serotonin, which helps prevent depression.

Water helps the production of melatonin, which is nature's sleep regulator: helping with sleep disorders. Lack of energy can be boosted by water, in that water generates electrical and magnetic energy in every body cell, providing a natural power boost.

Do I sound smart after all those big words? I could go on and on with the benefits of drinking water. Now here's the trick. Drink *ice* water. Really, really cold water.

My sister-in-law recently told me that she has been into drinking LOTS of water, and always had her water at room temperature, so that it was easier to 'gulp down.' She was missing out on some incredible caloric benefits. (You're gonna love this tip!)

When you drink ice water, your body uses energy to heat up the water to match the temperature of your body so that it can be used for hydration. The colder the water, the more energy it takes to heat it up.

According to the American Heart Association, the average person is supposed to consume about 64 oz. of water a day, or eight 8-oz. glasses. This averages to about 64 calories burned, depending on the temperature of the water and your body. The colder the water, the more calories you burn. Now isn't that FUN?! You're drinking a 0 calorie beverage that actually burns calories for you! Take it cold, my friends. The colder the better. Happy calorie burning!

Before going out to a gathering where you know there will be lots of food that you don't want to eat, drink a good amount of water beforehand. Now, in my opinion, party food (especially finger foods) are a pure delight, and so yummy. I could almost live on appetizers alone. Seriously, who doesn't love a mini pig-in-the-blanket! BUT if you are in the lose weight mode, and can't bear to splurge on a spread of appetizers, make sure you drink plenty of water (calorie-free!) beforehand and during the gathering.

The same trick goes for eating out at a restaurant. If you want to avoid eating too much— too many chips or too much bread, just keep sipping your water. It really does fill you up. Plus, drinking extra cold ice water during your meal puts you into that negative calorie mode. If you are full half way through your main course, stop eating. Take the rest home for lunch the next day.

There's nothing worse than going beyond your 'full limit' and feeling sickly stuffed. Eat slowly, drink lots of water, and you'll soon find that you can't finish the amount of food that you used to eat!

Chew Gum

What? I know, this seems like a weird one. Here's when to chew gum: when you're cooking or baking. I am probably the #1 abuser of the don't nibble while cooking or baking rule. That's the hidden beauty of baking cookies though, isn't it? Snacking on the dough? Oh, it's so good. I especially love brownie mix with chocolate chips. Cake batter? Yum. Frosting? Even yummier. See? This is part of my problem! I don't think about all the calories I am consuming while baking and cooking. A nibble here, and nibble there, and the calories add up.

Stick a piece of gum in your mouth. Having your mouth filled with calorie-free gum (especially mint flavored) will cut the desire to nibble on cookie dough and other delicious treats while cooking. Now, if you're determined enough to eat cookie dough, it won't be too difficult to take the gum out and stuff the dough in. But if you are serious about cutting calories, it's a good tip.

Fill Up On Negative Calorie Foods

Negative calorie foods? Really? Well, here's how this works. Below is a list of foods that (if eaten without dips and toppings) actually burn more calories in their digestion than they contain in their natural state. *So*, you can eat these foods with their natural amounts of calories, but those calories disappear when the body metabolizes them. Pretty much magical food.

See, I totally believe that God has created all the foods we need for healthy living and consumption. Eat away, my friends! Eat away and be skinny!

Here are the top negative calorie foods:

• Oranges
• Strawberries
• Grapefruit
• Carrots
• Apricots
• Lettuce
• Tomatoes
• Cucumbers
• Watermelon
• Apples
• Celery
• Tangerines
• Zucchini
• Cauliflower

Eat Breakfast

See, I told you some of these tips would seem

so simple. Eating breakfast is one of the best things you can do for losing weight. Research shows breakfast eaters are more successful at long-term weight loss than those who skip this meal. "It jump-starts your metabolism and prevents you from getting so ravenous you overeat later in the day," says Bonnie Taub-Dix, R.D., a New York City-based spokeswoman for the American Dietetic Association.

In a perfect world, I could eat one large bowl of Lucky Charms cereal every morning. I love Lucky Charms. I loved them as a child, and love them as an adult. Unfortunately, I don't think eating a bowl of them is the best way to lose weight...even though it does fall in line with the eat breakfast tip.

I've read that some super models eat only fruits in the morning up until noon. If you ate only the negative calorie fruits that I listed before, it would be as if you are jump starting your metabolism in the morning, and burning calories at the same time!

The single most important rule when it comes to breakfast for weight loss is: eat something. While a healthy, well-balanced meal is preferable, the truth is that you will be better off eating half a toasted bagel, a cereal bar or even a quick pastry than eating nothing at all.

By the time you get up in the morning, your

body has been without any food for at least six to eight hours, which means it is then running on fumes. If you don't have anything to eat in the first 60 minutes of being awake, your body will start burning off muscle tissue in order to feed itself. This will set off a cycle that will affect your glucose (blood sugar), causing you to crave more sugars (carbohydrates) throughout the day.

My favorite breakfast is a bowl of cereal with almond milk. We made the move to almond milk a few years ago. Whole (cow) milk is a bit gag-y to me now. Sorry to you whole milk drinkers out there. Almond milk with Special K cereal is my traditional breakfast. I think my liking towards just a bowl of cereal in the morning is one of the reasons I was never successful on the Atkins Diet. I was so tired of bacon and eggs that all I wanted was just *some cereal*.

Choose your breakfast items of choice. Now, I believe it is quite obvious that the consumption of donuts every day is not the wisest of breakfast choices. Eat, but be wise. Oatmeal, eggs, whole grain toast, fruit smoothies, plain fruit, breakfast bars, and healthy cereals are all great choices. Get your metabolism going, and enjoy something healthy to eat within the first sixty minutes of your morning.

Don't Deny Yourself

OK, so I understand that the reason that so much of America is obese and out of control weight-wise is because we have not denied ourselves when it comes to eating habits. It's true; we have become accustomed to grotesquely sized food portions, and no control in what we eat.

Don't get me wrong. I am not saying that a 'diet tip' is to eat whatever you want anytime you want. Unfortunately when you completely give up the foods you love, a person will tend to find something else to fill that food void. You will either fill that void with an unhealthy new habit, or you will deny yourself to the point to going slightly insane and end up eating unreal amounts of the food that you were trying to get away from!

Have you ever done that? Honestly? I have. I tried to do a period of no chocolate. Chocolate just happens to be my absolute weakness, and something in my system desires it. It really does. Wish it weren't true, but it is. So, when I thought to myself, *I will not eat anymore chocolate.* ALL I could think about was how much I wanted some. I went without chocolate consumption as long as I could. (Was it two days? Three?)

Finally I got to the point where I told myself, *Who cares? You're in charge of your own body. If you want chocolate, eat some chocolate!* Eat some

I did. I over did it. Then I could have used a shrink to deal with the feelings I had afterward. Couldn't find a free one, so I turned on Dr. Phil. That's what you get for free.

The moral of the above story? If you want some chocolate, have some. The key word here is *some*. If I can have a teensy snack of ten chocolate-chips, I find that I'm actually quite satisfied. A few chocolate chips won't destroy my figure. I feel satisfied that I have had my chocolate fix without going overboard calorie-wise. It's a win-win! Moderation is our weight loss friend.

Eat Slowly

Gotta be honest, this is not one of my favorite tips. It drives me crazy when I'm at a restaurant with a group, and there's that one person that everyone is sitting around waiting on to finish their meal. Come on! We have places to go and things to do!

Studies have actually shown that eating slower can help you lose weight! Just by eating slower, you'll consume fewer calories. Possibly even enough to lose twenty pounds a year by just eating slower. Sounds impossible, doesn't it?

Here's how it works. Your brain takes twenty minutes to register that the stomach is full. If we eat fast, we actually eat past the point of fullness, and by the time our brain registers 'full,' we are actually stuffed, and have eaten past the point of healthy fullness. If you take less bites and eat considerably slower, at the twenty minute mark, if we have eaten a proper amount of food, our brains (should) tell our bodies *stop eating, you are now full.*

The difficult part of this tip is to actually listen to our brains telling us to stop eating. I know many times when I feel full, and tell myself that I am good to go, the dessert menu comes around. "Did you all save room for desert?"

It all sounds and looks so good and we feel that we actually do have room left for dessert. After that dessert is when it starts to hurt. Cramped fullness. Bloated bellies. Ugh. If we had just listened to our bodies!

Did you know that there is actually a Slow Food Movement. (Those are some serious slow eaters!) A Slow Food Movement with its own Slow Food Manifesto. I won't be purchasing one of those manifestos anytime soon, but I will put into practice that wisdom of eating slower and listening to my brain tell me when I have had enough to eat.

Hopefully some of these tips will be helpful to you. Helpful towards making you the best you possible. I believe that God desires for us to thrive in body and spirit. It's all connected. What's happening on the inside is mirrored on the outer layers. I want to live my best. I want you to live your best, too.

FRUIT SALAD FACIAL

The previous chapter had some diet tips. This is the chapter for some beauty tips. I love this stuff. I've had such fun researching all kinds of goopy and unusual skin treatments. All for you. All for your skin.

My husband has had the pleasure of seeing me wear all sorts of lotions and concoctions on my face around the house. I need to apologize to him for some of the stinky face products I have applied right before bedtime. It's all for the book, Darling. For the book, and for you wonderful readers. After all of my experimenting, I now have some great skin tips. And, I have really tried them all for you.

I'll start off with some of my favorite finds. Top of the list (it's a simple one) is olive oil. Especially extra virgin olive oil, and yes, this is a chapter on beauty tips, not diet tips. This is an oldie but a goodie. I mean really old. The ancient Greeks and Egyptians used olive oil cosmetically for thousands of years.

Olive oil is a fatty acid and the skin needs fatty acids to keep it replenished and avoid drying out. As a fatty acid, olive oil also helps in cell rejuvenation. Olive oil is rich in vitamin E and vitamin A. Vitamin E gives you a youthful appearance by slowing aging. Vitamin A is what gives skin a healthy, natural glow.

Olive oil is also filled with antioxidants that fight free radicals that cause skin to age. Olive oil works well as an eye make-up remover. If you use olive oil daily, your skin will return to producing the oil it needs. Your skin will look smooth and radiant.

If using to remove make-up, just use a little dab, and it should do the trick. To moisturize, use a small amount, and massage into your skin. You can use another moisturizer on top, if you wish.

I have used olive oil on my face, and it really is wonderful. One of my new favorites, though, is to make a homemade body sugar scrub with olive oil. I mix regular white sugar, olive oil, and some peppermint essential oil, and it is wonderful to use at the end of your shower. I usually will slather/rub/scrub the mixture, then rinse, and towel dry. It's so refreshing, and honestly, the olive oil makes your skin look and feel wonderful! I highly recommend it!

Play around in your kitchen using olive oil as the base for a scrub. I also made one using almond extract and cocoa powder! Yum. It all rinses off easily in the shower, but the delightful scents will stay with you.

I do have to admit that one of the olive oil sugar scrubs I made didn't turn out so well. I have read that coffee grounds are great for the skin, and especially for cellulite. Caffeine's ability to increase circulation, even when applied topically, can get rid of water being stored in the body that can cause fat to be pushed against the skin, further aggravating the lumpy appearance.

Also, being a stimulant, caffeine can give the skin a more toned and firm appearance, similar to what is seen as a result of exercise. This effect also helps to reduce the appearance of cellulite.

Knowing this, I attempted to make a cellulite-reducing olive oil and sugar scrub. Bye, bye cellulite. The only problem is that the coffee grounds are tough to get off your skin, and seem to get everywhere in the shower. While the scrub smelled absolutely delicious, it was quite a mess. Perhaps you want to give coffee grounds a try. Do it! Just be prepared to find little grounds not wanting to be washed off your body.

Here's a rather unusual facial treatment. I know it sounds very odd, and a bit gross, but it works wonders. Preparation H cream. Yes, that's right. No typo here. I know this product is generally used 'down below,' but I'm telling you it works great on the face for smoothing out wrinkles.

'Preparation H's original formula includes shark liver oil and bio-dyne which is a group of substances that hasten sugar metabolism and encourage cellular reproduction and growth. Biodynes are also referred to as tissue and skin respiratory factors and today this compound is obtained from yeast and is known as Live Yeast Cell Derivatives. LYCDs contain minerals, carbohydrates, nucleic and amino acids and proteins and oxygenate skin tissues that hasten cell repair and growth and the FDA classifies LYCDs as wound healing agents.' –Website on Wrinkle Creams.

Preparation H for wrinkles is easy to use and for many results can be seen in a few weeks. Gently rubbing a small amount of cream under and around the eyes where bags, discoloration and wrinkles have appeared and allowing the cream to remain on the skin is the most effective way to use Preparation H. Patience and perseverance is important when waging war against wrinkles, it took time for wrinkles to form and it will take some time to reduce the severity and visibility of wrinkles.

Advocates of treating wrinkles with Preparation H state that using this cream twice a day everyday will produce results in two to four weeks depending on how deep the wrinkles are.

You can only get the original Preparation H in Canada. I ordered it over a month ago, and it was very easy to find and order online. It has made my skin so soft. It really is wonderful!

The only drawback is that you mildly smell like a fish market. To combat the odor, I applied a light non-fishy scented moisturizer on top of the Preparation H. Bingo. Scent gone, and still receiving the benefits. It took me a few days to come up with the additional moisturizer on top idea, so for those first days, my husband deserves a special award for dealing with the scent. Love you, honey.

Special note, after I bought and used the Canadian formula, I learned that there are skin benefits to the Prep H found in America, too. Apparently, the American formula is excellent for fast skin firming results. Apply the cream, and immediately your skin will appear firmer.

When you wash off the American Prep H, you also wash off the instantaneous results. The

Canadian cream is what works best for long-term wrinkle treatment. I happen to like the benefits that both formulas give. I'll be American during the day under my make-up for taunt skin, and be Canadian at night for long-lasting results. My international skin regimen. I feel so cutting edge.

I told you earlier that I've been putting all kinds of crazy stuff on my face. Here's another one, but I love this too! Pepto Bismal as a facial mask! I know, I know. First off, I need to tell you that your face won't be bright pink afterward. Although there will be just a slight glow, which I loved.

Pepto Bismal contains salicylic acid, which is a great exfoliator for skin, and is especially helpful in treating acne. Just as Pepto Bismal coats and soothes the stomach, it does the same for your skin. I don't have an acne problem right now, but I still love the pepto mask. The skin tightens nicely, and feels extremely smooth afterward. I even bought the cheaper store-brand version, and it worked just as well.

Want an amazing moisturizing mask? Don't go to the beauty products section of your store. Head straight to the isle for constipation medicine! Laugh now...your face will look amazing afterward!

Milk of Magnesia is your wonder mask. Milk of Magnesia contains magnesium hydroxide. This substance soaks up facial oil just as well as clay masks.

What I personally found when I used the Milk of Magnesia was that my skin was unbelievably moisturized and soft. Great results. Again, as with the Pepto Bismal, I used the store-brand, and it worked wonderfully! For a few dollars, you can have dozens of masks in one bottle. Pennies per mask. How fun it that?

Now, one of the best masks you'll ever put on your Face? I need a drum roll for this one. CAT LITTER! Seriously. It forms an absolutely amazing clay mask. You might think I'm kidding, but I honestly have a cat litter mask on my face this very second as I'm writing these words.

You need to buy the non-clumping 100% clay cat litter. It's usually the cheapest litter available. Unscented kitty litter is nothing more or less than clay grains, to be more specific, Bentonite (volcanic ash) clay. This is exactly the same clay that is used in clay masks you pay big money for when you buy it in a store or spa!

A bit of science: When you add water to kitty litter or Bentonite, the molecular structure changes and an electrical charge is produced. The clay starts to swell like a sponge and this electrical charge attracts toxins into the mixture and once they are drawn, they stick to the clay because of this charge.

Scoop out approximately a tablespoon of clay cat litter, and add enough water to moisten. Warm it in the microwave for 15 seconds. Mash the litter, and smooth it across your face and neck. Even if you just use the watery part, you will get a great result. Don't worry if you have clumps. That's fine.

Let the mask dry, and rinse off. I promise you, you will love the results. Seriously. One of the most amazing skin treatments EVER. Follow up with a great moisturizer on your skin!

If you have just a few extra minutes, grind the litter up in a blender (or smaller juice blender). The fine texture of the ground up litter will give you a smoother more 'spreadable' mask.

I've heard it said to not put anything on your skin that you wouldn't put in your mouth (other than the cat litter mask...). So, I looked into edible facial remedies. I tell you, God created some great food that is also so beneficial for our skin! You can snack and get great skin care at the same time! I love it!

One of the all-time best for snacking and skin? Avocados! They're like God's miracle food. Avocados are considered the world's miracle fruit (it's actually considered either a fruit or vegetable) because of its nutrient contents such as vitamin K, dietary fiber, potassium, folic acid, vitamin B6, vitamin C, vitamin E, copper, vitamin K, and potassium.

Avocados have been shown to help the prevention and fight against breast cancer, prostate cancer, as well as heart disease. Pretty unbelievable health benefits, not to mention how wonderful it is when made into guacamole!

So there's proof that eating avocado is beneficial to your health, but what about slathering it on your skin? The flesh of an avocado is amazing for soothing sunburnt skin, and all of the vitamin E is unbelievably moisturizing. I tried it myself. I bought an avocado, and slathered the pulp directly onto my face. I let it sit for about 15 minutes, and rinsed it off. My skin was so smooth and soft. All the vitamins that can be ingested are also beneficial on the skin. Absolutely wonderful. I highly recommend the treatment.

Want a snack and facial mask? Take the remaining pulp, and mix up your favorite guacamole recipe while your skin is receiving a deep treatment. Snacks and skin care. Who knew!

You say tomato, I say tomato. Tomatoes make an excellent skin treatment for everything from large pores and acne to rashes and more. Tomatoes have cooling elements to soothe raw skin, astringents to remove excess oil, and tons of vitamin C and A to brighten dull skin and restore its health.

Here's a thought: guacamole on the face. Avocado and tomato in the blender, and voila, facial dip that is incredible for your skin. A guacamole mask combines the astringent, blackhead-and oil- reducing benefits of tomatoes with the antiseptic and moisturizing properties of avocados. This super-rich mask also contains vitamin A, C and E, all of which are essential for healthy skin. Pass the chips, please.

Bananas are also amazing for the face, too! (I'm really into these snacking and skin care foods, aren't I?) I recently just learned that the inside of a banana peel is excellent for taking the itch and redness out of mosquito bites, and also poison ivy! We haven't had mosquitoes yet this year, but I will totally try this remedy on the next bites. I hate poison ivy, but now I have a delicious cure!

You probably already know that bananas are loaded with vitamins, and are truly a must-have fruit. I've just got to list some of these amazing benefits of bananas.

Stress: Potassium is a vital mineral, which helps normalize the heartbeat, sends oxygen to the brain and regulates your body's water-balance. When we are stressed, our metabolic rate rises, thereby reducing our potassium levels. These can be re-balanced with the help of a high-potassium banana snack.

Smoking. Bananas can also help people trying to give up smoking, as the high levels of Vitamin C, A1, B6, B12 they contain, as well as the potassium and magnesium found in them, help the body recover from the effects of nicotine withdrawal.

Strokes. According to research in The New England Journal of Medicine, eating bananas as part of a regular diet can cut the risk of death by strokes by as much as 40%!

Post Menstrual Syndrome. Forget the pills, and eat a banana. The vitamin B6 it contains regulates blood glucose levels, which can affect your mood.

Ulcers. The banana is used as the dietary food against intestinal disorders because of its soft texture and smoothness. It is the only raw fruit that can be eaten without distress in over-chronic ulcer cases. It also neutralizes over-acidity and reduces irritation by coating the lining of the stomach.

Morning Sickness. Snacking on bananas between meals helps to keep blood sugar levels up and avoid morning sickness.

Depression: According to a recent survey undertaken by MIND among people suffering from depression, many felt much better after eating a banana. This is because bananas contain tryptophan, a type of protein that the body converts into serotonin known to make you relax, improve your mood and generally make you feel happier.

The list goes on and on, but I think those are enough incentives to ingest bananas. Wanna get rid of a wart? Rub the inside of a banana peel on the wart for one to two weeks, and you should see results! The key compounds in the peel include potassium and other antioxidants that help to keep the skin looking soft, supple and healthy.

I've just been learning all these wonderful tips. How come I didn't hear of all of these when I was younger? That's OK, now we all will know some unbelievable uses for bananas.

So while you're munching on a banana to ward off PMS pangs, take a quarter of it, mash it up, and slather it on your face. I tried this once without mashing it well, and it was quite lumpy. Take the additional seconds to mash the fruit with a fork, and the smoother consistency will be a lot easier to keep on your face.

Your face will feel firm and smooth, and the anti-aging properties are extremely beneficial. Want an extra moisturizing mask? Add some honey in with your banana.

Warning: you may not want to be dressed up while applying and wearing these two ingredients. Be in your sweats of pajamas in case of drippage! Don't worry if it drips in your mouth, it's actually quite yummy!

You're so gonna love me for this next edible skin care fruit. One of my favorite fruits is the strawberry. Mix up some cream cheese with sugar as a dip for them, and this girl is in Heaven. But, I have lived my whole life (until this previous year) not knowing how beneficial strawberries can be for your skin— especially skin with acne. Strawberries are also listed in those negative calorie foods (minus the cream cheese dip), so it makes them even better!

Seriously, all you have to do is slice a strawberry and rub it all over your face. The salicylic acid in the strawberry will naturally treat the acne, and just naturally exfoliate your face!

Again, you are so very welcome! Nibble, rub on face, nibble, treat acne. What a wonderful world we live in! If you just want to enjoy the exfoliating benefits of the natural salicylic acid, but don't need to treat acne, try this wonderful strawberry and sour cream mask.

Seriously, friends, it just doesn't get any better than this! Blend half cup of strawberries with one tablespoon of sour cream. Stir the mixture well and apply on your skin.

Keep the mask on your skin for twenty minutes and then wash it off with lukewarm water. The strawberries in the mixture will help to tighten and soothe your skin while the cream eliminates out all the dirt and dead cells from the skin. This remedy also moistens your skin.

Do you have large pores? Fear not, I have another edible fruit skin enhancer. Oranges. That's right, delicious, juicy oranges that are loaded with vitamin C, antioxidants, and yet again, salicylic acid.

Not too many years ago, the beauty industry came out with 'miracle creams' that contained vitamin C. Remember? First there were alpha hydroxy acids, then moisturizers with salicylic acid, then vitamin C, then all the retinol products. Well, everyone knows that oranges are loaded with natural vitamin C. The beauty of that? Just apply the natural juice of an orange on to your face, and you will have the same benefits and results as with a hundred dollar cream!

If you want to shrink facial pores, take out juice from one orange and apply it directly on your face like a face wash and then rinse immediately. The Vitamin C in the orange juice will add smoothness and softness to your skin instantly.

Orange juice is also considered very efficient in shrinking enlarged pores. All you have to do is dip a cotton ball in orange juice completely, and apply it to the enlarged pores. Leave it for 2 to 3 minutes and then rinse it. Simple. Sip, tone your skin, sip, shrink your pores. Lovely.

Using an expensive toner at home? You can use orange juice as a great skin toner. It also helps your skin from damage from the sun. Simply rub half of an orange or Clementine all over the face. Leave it on for 5 minutes. Rinse with cold water in the end and experience a beautiful, fresh and glowing skin in a jiffy. This is so fun, isn't it?

As with strawberries, oranges are also fantastic in acne treatment. Orange juice acts as a natural astringent and helps a great deal to dry up your zits. Regular use of oranges in your beauty routine also helps to prevent your skin from acne and blemishes. At the same time the fruit acids in orange juice also exfoliate your skin lightly.

Honestly, I hope you're having as much fun reading this chapter as I am writing it. I'm getting hungry for fruit salad, and ready to sit with some honey and banana on my face! Snacking and skincare. Two of my all-time favorite things.

Experiment with different vegetables and fruits on your face. Really! Pineapple will work just as great as the oranges and strawberries! Blend fruits with whole cream.

Cream and milk have been recognized and used in beauty regiments for thousands of years! Milk contains lactic acid and what this does is act as a gentle exfoliator, removing dead outer skin cells and helping reveal new soft ones.

Milk also soothes the skin and is very gentle. Using skim milk though, is not as useful as the whole fat milk. If you're going whole milk, you might as well use real cream. Strawberries and cream, oh yum.

To be honest with you, I might have a slight difficulty saving enough of my treat to put on my face. Decisions, decisions.

Now I'm hungry.

THE BEST KEPT BEAUTY SECRET

I truly hope that this book has been beneficial to you. I really do. We only have one chance to walk through this life, and I so desire for you to walk through it in a completely fulfilling fashion.

I wish you deep joy, happiness, health, and peace. Strive to be all that God created you to be. Live out your dreams. Don't give up on goals.

Yesterday at the gym, it dawned on me that being at my best physically is still an achievable goal. The body can still be molded and shaped, no matter what age. It's also that way with your dreams and goals.

If you always wanted to be a pianist, it's not too

late. Whatever career or personal goal that you may have given up on is still an option in your life. It's still a possibility. Don't give up on, or forget your dreams.

We were in the Phoenix airport not too long ago, and they had a huge billboard for the University of Arizona showing a ninety-two year old woman that had just received her diploma. She was absolutely adorable in her cap and gown.

I love that. It's never too late. Even at ninety-two this woman was starting a new career. How inspirational!

Perhaps you think that getting in shape, or being 'beautiful' is what someone else can attain, not you. Perhaps you've been told your whole life that you aren't as pretty as the other girls, or that you could never be a size 6. Don't believe it. You hold the power to still become who you want to become.

There have been enough shows on TV about people at every age, and at every weight getting themselves healthy, and perfectly fit.

Do you remember the TV show The Swan. Now, some people thought it was controversial to make someone completely over, including tummy tucks and surgeries. I thought it was wonderful to see the transformations. Some of these women were literally called ugly their whole lives, through the transformations on the show, were absolutely stunning. It can happen. It can happen to you, if you so desire.

Never think it's too late. Never give up. I know surgeries, tummy tucks, Botox and other injections are sometimes thought of as taboo, especially in the Christian world. *Be happy with how God made you* is a familiar thought. I've got to be honest, if you have the money, and a tummy tuck is what you've always wanted after having all your children, then more power to you. If I had the extra cash, I'd love to have the fat sucked out of my thighs and stomach!

I just don't want you to feel that it is wrong to get some help with your body or wrinkles. It's *your* body. You should feel good in your own skin.

Don't worry about other people's opinions. (Well, except maybe the opinion of your spouse...). Make the most out of the life you are given, stand tall and beautiful. You deserve it.

Solomon has some great additional verses in Proverbs to add to the ones I presented in earlier chapters. *"Souls who follow their hearts thrive; fools bent on evil despise matters of soul."* Proverbs 13:19

This verse reflects my feelings towards you living life at its best, and not giving up on your dreams. Follow your heart. When you are following your heart, you are filled with joy and happiness. Joy and happiness are then reflected from your heart to your countenance.

I never get tired of people watching. I thoroughly enjoy it. Perhaps that is one of the reasons I enjoy traveling so much. It gives me the opportunity to observe so many different kinds of people. People at malls and airports are the best. Perhaps it's the wanna-be psychologist in me, but I love watching and trying to figure out people.

In my opinion, the majority of people don't look happy. So many look tired, worn, and defeated. I'm reading all of that from their faces and demeanor. And, yes, a majority of Christians look that same exact way. It's unfortunate, but true.

I don't want someone to look at my face and body language, and 'read' me as a defeated woman. I count it a huge blessing that I absolutely love what I am able to do for my career. Speaking, singing, and writing brings fulfillment.

I am happy when I am using my gifts and able to bring in paychecks from doing what I love. I also believe that reflects on my face. I truly do. Doing what I love to do in life is also beneficial to my health.

"A cheerful disposition is good for your health; gloom and doom leave you bone-tired." Proverbs

17:22

See why I want you to walk fulfilled? It's good for you! The inward and outward have a symbiotic relationship. Do you remember the term symbiosis from beginning biology? "A symbiotic relationship is a relationship between two entities which is mutually beneficial for the participants of the relationship. Thus there is a positive-sum gain from cooperation.

This is a term commonly used in biology to explain the relationship between two entities that need each other to survive and prosper. The bumblebee and the flower would be an example. The bumble bee extracts the flower's pollen for protein and its nectar for energy. The bumblebee, while collecting these sources, inadvertently brushes pollen from one flower to another to ensure the flower's reproduction process begins. The bumblebee needs the flower to survive; the flower needs the bumblebee to survive." (BiologyOnline.org)

In order for your outer appearance to look good, you need to be thriving and full of life on the inside. They go hand in hand. They need each other.

You may have the perfect body and made-up face, but if you are unhappy in your heart, it will show. All the make-up in the world can't disguise a sad heart and spirit.

Your health is depending upon your inner joy, also. *"Gloom and doom leave you bone tired."* I've been bone tired before. There's a difference between good and bad bone tired, though.

A few weeks ago we had excessive rain, which led to flooding in our basement. After five days of continuous hard rain, the ground around our home was saturated, and there was nowhere else for the rain to go, but in our house. In fact, it was Easter Sunday evening, of all days!

I had gone to Walmart (I know, I know...on Easter Sunday night, ugh) to buy some food and supplies. My husband called me and said, "Hurry, buy a wet vac and get home; the basement is flooding!" Not the best of calls.

I bought a 4.5 gallon wet vac (which I later realized was extremely too small) and headed home. Our pastor came to our rescue with two 16 gallon wet vacs, and we sucked up and dumped water (16 gallons of water is heavy!) for twelve straight hours.

By 7:30 Monday morning, the incoming water had slowed enough that we could just throw down some towels, and sleep for a few hours. That afternoon around 3pm, the rain and flooding started again. We sucked and dumped water until 2am.

That next day, I could honestly say that I was 100% bone tired. Exhausted. Not a good bone tired, either.

A good bone tired? The complete and utter exhaustion a mother feels after giving birth to a child. You couldn't be more tired, but it's a *good* tired. What a beautiful reward for some of the hardest physical labor you will ever experience.

I have a feeling that Proverbs 17:22 is referring to bone tiredness that people experience when they are filled with negativity and an outlook of despair. No thank you.

If you are reading this book and you feel that you are a person living with a defeated soul, I encourage you to rise above it. If you don't have a personal relationship with Jesus, your Creator and Savior, it is my heart's desire that you would accept him to come into your heart to take away your guilt and despair.

And in asking him to be Lord of your whole life, that he would fill you with a joy that you never thought possible, peace beyond your wildest dreams, and a new hope for your future. It is possible, and it's so fulfilling. A total renewing of your spirit is probably the best beauty advice I can give you.

Your face will change, you will glow and shine in a way you never thought possible. *"A cheerful* heart brings a smile to your face; a sad heart makes it hard to get through the day." Proverbs 15:13. "The wage of a good person is exuberant life; an evil person ends up with nothing but sin." Proverbs 10:16

The benefits of having a relationship with Jesus and making Him first in your life are innumerable. Having a cheerful God-filled heart will bring a true beautiful smile to your face, and you will experience exuberant life. Believe me, even the most expensive beauty creams can't give you results like that! Plus, there's no monetary expense. It's a win-win.

There's even more. This is one of my favorite promises: "A twinkle in the eye means joy in the heart, and good news makes you fit as a fiddle." Proverbs 15:30

I love that wording, and it's so entirely true. I'm attracted to people that have a twinkle in their eye. They're happy people. This verse reinforces my belief that what is on the inside shines through on the outside. Joy in your heart 'twinkles' through your eyes, and I believe eyes that twinkle are beautiful eyes.

Apparently people that seek after God's ways are also fit as fiddles when they hear good news, too. It just keeps getting better! Aren't these great verses! They're so encouraging and so full of great beauty wisdom.

I honestly believe that if you follow the teachings of all the scripture references I quoted in this book, and take the steps for a healthy and beautiful you on the inside and out, you won't ever need to buy another book on beauty. I know that's a high claim to make, but I believe it 100%.

Now, you may buy new books on make-up application. Make-up trends change all the time, but beauty is timeless. Some of the beauty tips in this book have been in use for thousands of years. Those are truly time tested!

Follow after these wise scriptures, and walk fulfilled in your life's calling. Be who God created you to be. Don't settle for living less than your full potential. Your inner joy will radiate through you, and people will notice your beauty. The beauty that comes from being the best you possible.

YOUR FACE IS SO YUMMY!

I thought it would be fun to give you a bunch of recipes for facial masks. Have fun experimenting with these recipes, or be creative, and mix up some of your very own concoctions. The world of facial masks is yours. Enjoy!

Easy Anti-Aging Mask
1 tsp of honey
A few drops of orange juice.

Preparation
1. Mix the two together well.
2. Spread mixture over entire face even around the eyes and mouth.
3. Leave it on for 20 minutes if possible, and then

remove with lots of warm water and a pad of cotton.

*This mixture is especially good for mature skin and will put softness into younger skins which have been over dried by wind or sun. If used regularly it can stave off those fine lines that appear as we get older.

Aspirin Face Mask

Dissolve 3-4 coated Aspirins in a few drops of mild water.

Add more water if needed until you get a mix that can be applied on the face.

Let it rest for 15 minutes (until it dries and undissolved pieces start to fall off).

Rinse off with lukewarm water using a washcloth.

(Be careful so that it doesn't get into your eyes!)

This mask is recommended for all skin types, although it shows best effects on oily skin and skin prone to acne, Its and blackheads. Apply this mask no more than twice a month.

Natural Face-Lift Mask

2 egg yolks
1 teaspoon of sugar

Preparation :
Whisk the egg yolks until the mass is firm and consistent.
Add sugar gradually and mix well to combine the two.
Apply on the face and leave on for 25 minutes.
Wash off with warm water using a wash cloth.

Strawberry Mask
1/2 cup of strawberry
1/4 cornstarch

Preparation:
Mix strawberries and cornstarch together to make a paste. Apply to face. Leave for 30 minute rinse off with cool water.

Apple and Cinnamon Mask
1 large apple (peeled, cleaned and grated)
1/2 teaspoon of whipped cream
1 teaspoon of honey
1 tablespoon of oatmeal
1/2 teaspoon of cinnamon

Preparation:
Mix all the ingredients until the mass starts looking like a paste.
Apply on the face and leave on for 10 minutes.

Gently rub the face to enhance the exfoliating properties of oatmeal.

Rinse off with cold water and gently dry off with a towel.

Chocolate Face Mask
1/3 cup cocoa
1/4 cup of honey
2 tablespoons of heavy cream (sour cream will work as well)
3 teaspoons of oatmeal powder

Preparation:
Mix all the ingredient until the mass in consistent. Apply on the face, gently massaging it so that oatmeal can start exfoliating the dead skin cell layer. Leave it on for about 15 to 20 minutes and rinse off with lukewarm water.

Carrot Facial Mask
2-3 large carrots
4 1/2 tablespoons honey

Preparation:
Cook carrots, then mash. Mix with honey. Apply gently to the skin and wait 10 minutes. Rinse off with cool water.

Cream Cheese and Carrot Face Mask
1 medium size carrot
2 tablespoons of cream cheese

Preparation:
Mash a carrot. Use 2 tablespoons of it. Mix with a tablespoon of cream cheese. Apply to face and neck. After 15 min rinse the face off water.

Egg white mask
1 egg white
1 teaspoon of honey
1 teaspoon of olive oil
1 teaspoon of lemon juice

Preparation:
Combine all the ingredients into a smooth paste and apply on the previously cleansed face and neck. Leave on for 25 minutes and rinse well.

Kiwi Skin Firmer
1 ripe kiwi (peeled)
1 teaspoon of honey

Preparation:
Mix the kiwi in a blender or mash with a fork if it is soft. Strain the excess liquid (juice) and add the teaspoon of honey. Apply the mass on the face and leave on for 20 minutes. Rinse off with warm water.

Cherry Natural Face Lift
30 ripe cherries (remove the pits)
2 tablespoons of honey

Preparation:
Blend the cherries in a blender or mash them if they are ripe enough. Add honey and combine the two.

(I didn't mention cherries in the previous chapter of yummy ingredients for facial masks. When you think of cherries, the first thing that comes to mind is a cherry pie. But, it can be used as a very efficient mask that firms the skin's top layer and diminishes the appearance of wrinkles and lines. Its red pigment is also a powerful antioxidant.)

Grapefruit Facial Mask
1 teaspoon grapefruit juice
1 teaspoon sour cream

1 egg white

Preparation:
This is for an oily to normal skin type. Beat egg white until it is fluffy, add sour cream and grapefruit juice and blend well. Apply to face for 15 minutes, then rinse with warm water.

Fountain of Youth Facial Mask
2 teaspoon sour cream
1/2 teaspoon honey
1/2 teaspoon lemon juice
3 capsules vitamin E

Preparation:
Mix together all of the ingredients in a bowl. Apply to your face and neck avoiding the eye area. Leave on for 10 to 15 minutes. Rinse off this facial mask with lukewarm water.

About The Author

Kirsten Hart has been able to travel with some of America's premier Christian singing groups, including The Spurrlows, FRIENDS (the back-up group for Grammy Award winner Larnelle Harris), The Richard Roberts TV Singers, and as a Praise and Worship Leader for Benny Hinn Crusades as well as on TBN's This Is Your Day telecast.

She has had the amazing opportunity to sing on television, in hundreds of churches, and as part of international crusades. She has shared her heart before thousands. She also counts it a privilege to have sung for FOCUS ON THE FAMILY and COMPASSION INTERNATIONAL events, Camp Meetings, Statewide Conventions, and more.

Kirsten has spoken in churches and for Women's Ministry Events across the country for the past twenty years. Recently, God chose to give her a new life story in a surprising way. As she is daily walking out her story, she brings a message of grace, forgiveness, and miracles!

Kirsten is available to share her story, as well as other keynote topics for churches, retreats, and conferences. She is the author of three CHAT Bible studies, as well as *ReInventing You/Regenerate Your Life,* and her story, *Baby Girl Murphy/Alias Identity.*

Visit her website: www.kirstenhart.com for more details.

ALSO AVAILABLE ON AMAZON.COM

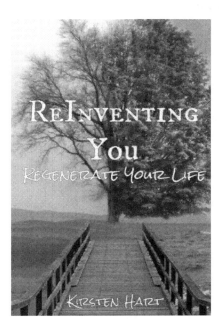

Queen Esther was just an ordinary Hebrew girl that God reinvented into a Queen in order to save His people. King David was reinvented from a shepherd boy to a King. Moses was 80 when he was called to lead the nation of Israel.

What does God have yet in store for your life? Explore the possibilities that God has for you in every changing season of your journey.

Newlywed to young mom to empty nester to retirement age--God can transform your life at every stage to use your gifts in ways greater than you could ever imagine. There are no limits to how God can reinvent your life to maximize all of your potential.

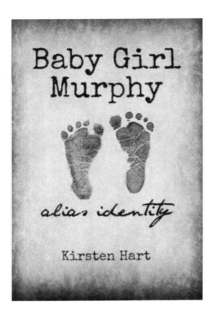

"I'm sorry, Mrs. Hart, we don't have any birth records for you."
These were the words I heard over the phone when I was trying to
locate a copy of my birth certificate for a new passport. "Have you
checked with the Adoption Registry Office?" was the following
question. Adoption? I was forty-one years old. I knew who my
parents were. Why would someone suggest that I talk with an
Adoption Registry Office? I just simply needed a copy of my birth
certificate. That phone call led me on a new journey of discovery
and secrets.

Who was I? Who was my birth mother? Did I have other siblings?
What was my story? Baby Girl Murphy is my personal exploration of
discovering my new identity and unveiling a secret that God had
kept for 41 years. A secret so dear, yet so mysterious. "...Find out
more..." were the words I kept hearing echo through my heart.
Indeed I did find out more. More than I ever dreamed imaginable.

WWW.AMAZON.COM

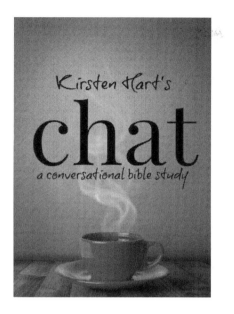

CHAT is for every small group that enjoys digging into intriguing Biblical topics. Set aside time to grab some snacks and coffee, and journey into a Bible study that seeks to draw out conversations whether in a living room or neighborhood café.

This is not your average small group study. CHAT contains twelve individual topics that aren't successive, yet can be used on a weekly basis. Pick and choose. Jump around. It's up to you.

Designed for busy people with an appetite for truth, and connection with each other and God.

WWW.AMAZON.COM

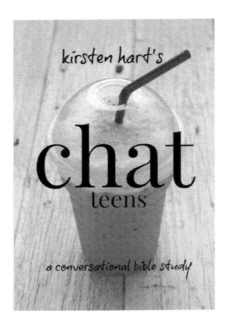

CHAT is for every teen group that enjoys digging into intriguing Biblical topics. Set aside time to grab some snacks and a cappuccino, and journey into a Bible study that seeks to draw out conversations whether in a living room or neighborhood café.

This is not your average small group study. CHAT contains twelve individual topics that aren't successive, yet can be used on a weekly basis. Pick and choose. Jump around. It's up to you. Designed for busy teens with an appetite for truth, and connection with each other and God.

*CHAT Teens is the teen version of CHAT for adults—(the red cup cover). CHAT Teens contains the same chapter topics as the adult version (except for one chapter) just worded for the teen audience. Teens and their parents can dig in, and discuss the same Bible topics at home!

WWW.AMAZON.COM

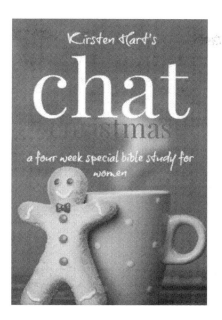

CHAT Christmas is a special edition of the CHAT 'A Conversational Bible Study' series. Usually the CHAT books contain twelve separate chapters. This Christmas edition only contains four, and is meant as a special study to fit in-between Thanksgiving and Christmas. Designed to concentrate on this time of celebrating Thanksgiving and the birth of our Lord.

CHAT was designed not to be a right or wrong answer conversational Bible study. No questions to fill in. And if you miss a week, you can't get behind. Every week has a non-chronological different topic of discussion. Grab a cup of coffee, a snack, and dig into challenging topics with your small group.

WWW.AMAZON.COM

Kirsten Hart

Made in the
USA
Lexington, KY